Aussie Midwives

Fiona McArthur has worked as a rural midwife for many years. She is a clinical midwifery educator, mentors midwifery students, and is involved with obstetric emergency education for midwives and doctors from all over Australia.

Fiona's love of writing has seen her sell over two million books in twelve languages. She is the author of the nonfiction works *The Don't Panic Guide to Birth* and *Breech Baby: A Guide for Parents*.

She lives on an often-swampy farm in northern New South Wales with her husband, Ian. She's constantly taking photographs of the sunrise and sunset and loves that researching her books allows her to travel to remote places.

fionamcarthurauthor.com

Aussie Midwives

FIONA McARTHUR

MICHAEL JOSEPH
an imprint of
PENGUIN BOOKS

MICHAEL JOSEPH

UK | USA | Canada | Ireland | Australia
India | New Zealand | South Africa | China

Penguin Books is part of the Penguin Random House group of companies
whose addresses can be found at global.penguinrandomhouse.com.

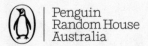

Penguin
Random House
Australia

First published by Penguin Group (Australia), 2016

Cover Design by Grace West © Penguin Group (Australia)
Cover images: midwife by Michelle Hamze; hospital interior by
Jose Juan Garcia/Getty Images; back cover landscape by Priscilla Turner.
Text Design © Penguin Group (Australia)
Typeset in Sabon, 12pt/18pt by Penguin Books (Australia)
Colour separation by Splitting Image Colour Studio, Clayton, Victoria
Printed and bound in Australia by Griffin Press, an accredited
ISO AS/NZS 14001 Environmental Management Systems printer.

National Library of Australia
Cataloguing-in-Publication data:

McArthur, Fiona, author.
Aussie midwives / Fiona McArthur.
9780143799993 (paperback)
Midwives–Australia–Anecdotes.
Midwifery–Australia–Anecdotes.

618.200922

penguin.com.au

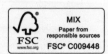

To passionate midwives and powerful mothers
With love

Contents

Introduction   *1*

1   **A rural midwife**   7
    Fiona McArthur

2   **Grassroots midwifery**   16
    Rae Condon

3   **The negotiator and breech**   30
    Kate Braye

4   **Small-town midwife**   42
    Lisa Ferguson

5   **First-year midwife**   48
    Bronwyn Thomas

6   **Midwife with wings**   60
    Jillian Thurlow

7   **Emergency retrievals**   74
    Priscilla Turner

8   **Remote island midwife**   84
    Annie Delaine

9   **President, Australian College of Midwives**   102
    Caroline Homer

10 **From Alice to Katherine**   113
    Glenda Gleeson

11 **Coming home again**   124
    Hannah Dahlen

12 **Quest for safety**   138
    Mandy Hunter

13 **Women's business**   152
    Louise Paul

14 **Phone a PAL**   173
    Helen Cooke

15 **Birth at home**   182
    Shea Caplice

16 **High-risk pregnancy**   193
    Kate Dyer

17 **Nurturing neighbours**   208
    Heather Gulliver

18 **Baby whisperer**   220
    Michael Dixon

19 **From midwife to mother**   229
    Devon Plumley

    Acknowledgements   *243*

Introduction

In Australia, midwives care for women and families from the cities to the red centre and in every direction to the sea – so, in this, all our midwifery journeys are different. Being present as the midwife at a baby's birth is one of life's glorious adventures and an ongoing emotional journey. Australian midwives have incredible stories to share and they deal with different challenges, joys and heartbreaks – just like the mothers and families they serve.

In these pages, different midwives have been persuaded to tell their stories and share a window into their worlds. Collating this, my heart has been squeezed and my mind broadened with new insights. Even after thirty years as a midwife I'm shaking my head in awe. I am indeed privileged to have the opportunity to share these stories with you.

So what is a midwife and what is her scope of practice? From the International Confederation of Midwives 2011:

> The midwife is recognised as a responsible and accountable professional who works in partnership with women to give

the necessary support, care and advice during pregnancy, labour and the postpartum period, to conduct birth on the midwife's own responsibility and to provide care for the newborn and the infant. This care includes preventative measures, the promotion of normal birth, the detection of complications in mother and child, the accessing of medical care or other appropriate assistance and the carrying out of emergency measures.

The midwife has an important task in health counselling and education, not only for the woman, but also within the family and the community. This work should involve antenatal education and preparation for parenthood and may extend to women's health, sexual or reproductive health and childcare.

A midwife may practise in any setting including the home, community, hospitals, clinics or heath units.

Did I hear you say, 'That's a pretty big task'? Well, it is, but it is also a life-enriching career. Midwifery is on the brink of becoming a separate profession from general nursing, distinct from the more medicalised viewpoint that birthing women are patients. Midwives need different tools, because most pregnancies aren't about disease; they're about healthy women doing what they're inherently built to do – birth babies. A lot of the time midwifery is about sitting back and encouraging the woman to believe in herself, while providing the safe environment for her to do what she's designed to do. Which is why many midwives today train solely as midwives without merging with the world of the generalist nurse. A midwife's dream is that every birthing woman would see how incredible she is, how she is the central figure everyone else revolves around, and how in awe her midwife is as she watches over her. Midwives recognise fear has no place in birthing – it is the single most destructive emotion in a woman's birth space – and if an entering person carries fear they need to leave it outside the door or not come into the room.

Midwives need to be watchful, aware of danger signals and risk, but have the skill to deal appropriately with curve balls as they come. That's why we have ongoing education and drills and teamwork. During labour, everything needs to be about the woman in the birth space and everyone believing in her.

The new wave of young midwives from the universities are amazing, confident, passionate, zealous and sometimes a little quick to accept risk, but that comes with the territory. And they have stories too. They are taught to be autonomous and to question everything, to ensure practices are based on research and not followed just because we've always done it that way, and their passion makes me proud. Student midwives in universities in Australia read and hear about how it is when women embark on childbearing, and then they go into large hospitals full of high-tech equipment (tertiary hospitals), or small rural hospitals like mine, or somewhere in the middle of these extremes to learn their craft of being with women alongside registered midwives. They do hours in antenatal clinics, birthing, postnatal and caring for newborns. I love my new job as an educator, one of those helping students and new graduate midwives settle into the reality outside of uni and the joy of rural midwifery, as well as helping experienced midwives keep up with the rapid changes, but it's always a bonus when the ward is too busy and I have an opportunity to do what I've been doing for the last thirty years – sharing a woman's birthing as her midwife.

Some midwives in this book work from high-risk birth suites in huge tertiary hospitals where women are likely to have fewer choices because of special health factors. The team caring for them might include obstetricians, paediatricians, physicians and many other specialists but a critical care midwife can still create moments for the birthing woman and her at-risk baby that facilitate peace and power in the highly structured environment around them.

Outside of the hospital walls, the midwife takes on many responsibilities for women birthing at home or seeking care through a birthing centre, where the family has set their own stage, created their own plan, and built trust with their personal midwife to facilitate the birth in an environment and way they choose.

Early on in these chapters we wil also see midwifery through the eyes of a newly graduated midwife, fresh from university, fresh from the continuity women whom she followed through pregnancy, her mind full of research articles and snippets of experience, taught to be woman-centred and independent. Often these fledgling midwives find themselves in a hospital system that isn't always geared that way, because the old ways still exist, yet they find the magic of midwifery is brightly there, beckoning them to the future.

We will meet midwives who have worked in war-torn countries, or third-world and isolated work settings: from the more traditional concepts of small country town midwifery to the RFDS emergency midwives, the outback clinic midwives and even a midwife on the island of Saibai past Australia's most northern tip, and another in New Guinea teaching young PNG midwives how to save mothers' lives.

So join me as we visit midwives working in different models in different places in Australia – but all with the same mantra: to welcome your babies and be with women in pregnancy, birth and beyond.

CHAPTER 1

A rural midwife

Fiona McArthur

Babies often come quickly at the end.

In novels, the first thing focused on after a birth is the cry of the new baby. In real life, sometimes it's the sound of a first-time father hitting the floor and his camera skidding across the tiles. Dads don't get a lot of attention, because everyone else is busy up the business end, and no matter how many classes a couple may attend together, birth is usually more intense than they ever dreamed. In case you're worried about that dad, he was fine – a little sheepish, but a hero to me because he cared so much that he fainted. So even though we all know how it works, you never know what to expect when someone is having a baby.

I've always worked in my small rural hospital with about 300 births a year, though I'm also privileged to volunteer in obstetric education with like-minded doctors and midwives from across the country. In our hospital we only book in low-risk women, because we don't have specialist paediatricians or obstetricians on hand, but it's not unusual to have an unexpected breech baby pop out in the middle of the night or a set of 28-week twins decide they're not waiting for a CareFlight helicopter to come and retrieve their mother first.

We're good at managing until help arrives in the next hour or two, or six, and our caesarean birth rate is low. By we, I mean the midwives and the three multi-skilled local doctors who practise obstetrics along with everything else in GP land, and do most of the on-call medical roster.

For me, working rurally is a joy. It's not unusual to have been there for the birth of the mother herself, or even when both parents of this new baby were born. Some women fly in the door, push out their baby and go home four hours later because they prefer to rest with their families. Other mothers stay for days; sometimes the dads stay too, while mum and baby perfect their breastfeeding or savour the peace.

The best scenario is when you see a woman in antenatal clinic and parenting classes, then support her through labour, settle mother and baby into their room afterwards and are there the next day as the parents give that first baby bath. Later you have the pleasure of waving goodbye on discharge, with Dad carrying the baby and a displaced first child hanging on to their mother's hand. There's a lot of job satisfaction in that.

You may have guessed I love being a midwife. I love watching women become mothers. And I love watching student midwives become registered midwives. Because I live in a small community, I often meet children whose first moments I've witnessed, perhaps even helped them with that first breath if they were having a hard time, or worried over them when they became sick.

For all the many, many times that I meet a woman's eyes with the memory of a happy birth between us – whether we end up laughing about the fact her husband fainted straight away, or reminiscing about the baby's looks – there are the other times too.

Two years ago I ran into a mother at the supermarket checkout, amid the wrestle of the shopping trolleys on a day off. I couldn't remember her name, but I knew there'd been a baby between us. Then she said, very simply, 'It's a year today.' And I remembered. I'd been terrified the first time I'd listened to her baby's heartbeat, and we'd rushed mum directly to theatre. Later we'd transferred this fragile newborn via ambulance to a higher-level care facility. Nothing worked.

This mother and I share a bond that has nothing to do with her education, or her home life, or her job; what's between us is deeper and sadder.

In my other life I write deeply happy books, novels that I hope can soothe a stressed or broken heart. The happiness I weave into my books comes from knowledge of the good and the sad that's at the heart of every midwife's job. We are the guardians of the joyful and the broken-hearted.

It's a huge privilege to stand at the bedside of a labouring woman, to help her in a moment that she'll remember for the rest of her life. I'm the fortunate midwife who catches those wizened little creatures, with their screwed-up faces and blue fingers, their squalling voices and thrashing limbs. Or the sleek and sleepy baby that comes into the world serene.

But I'm also the one who leaves the room so that a mother and father can spend a moment, or an hour, or a day and night, with a child who is leaving them far too soon. A child who will never dance up to me in the grocery store and be introduced: 'Look, Molly. This lady helped me give birth to you.'

Some Mollys and Jacksons and Chrises dance off to other places. But they are loved, fiercely, for the time they are on earth. And I'm privileged to be there for that time as well.

Women are incredible. Very early in my working life, I met Joan, a woman who inspired my faith in the strength of birthing women. Joan was a first-time mum and the first woman I attended who wanted to birth on a mat on the floor with a beanbag to lean back on.

We had a new midwife in our tiny country maternity ward at this time. Her name was Hope, and she was red-haired and fierce when defending women. Hope was young, with radical ideas for the early eighties – ideas like birthing in a position the mother wanted, whether kneeling on the floor, standing up, or in the shower – and she had begun teaching the antenatal classes, and spreading the word to mums. The older midwives were sceptical, and shook their heads with predictions of dropped babies and broken backs for the carers. We young ones were wide-eyed and impressed by Hope's fearless defence of women's choice.

This day Joan, my allocated labouring woman, didn't want anything to do with lying on the bed. The older midwives happily passed her to me; newfangled ideas go with young midwives. It was 'Watch out for your back, and don't expect the doctor to get down there and deliver that baby.'

I was happy, Joan was happy, but her husband, a frowning, bleak worrier with a weak stomach that threatened to unman him at any moment, was very stressed. His face the colour of milk, he teetered on the edge of fainting, but he doggedly stayed and tried to be supportive. There was obvious love between them, but he was out of his comfort zone, a miserable pale cloud in the corner.

She ignored him. Joan had this. She blocked out his stress and was calm and confident, breathing quietly, shifting her position as she needed. I watched and absorbed her inherent knowledge – the way she tuned into her own body, shifting it every time it told her to move. I listened to her instinct and assisted when she needed me to. I loved her quiet breathing, her ease at being naked labouring in the shower despite being a very private person, her pure serenity and power.

The labour progressed, and she birthed with control and grace and a splash of water as her poor husband moaned. He wasn't going to be one of those men who rip off their shirt and cradle their naked wife and baby with tears running down their face, but he stayed, awed, and you knew that family had a future.

Afterwards, Joan rested back against the beanbag and we were silent with the wonder of it until I turned to the husband

and asked him if he'd be able to cut the umbilical cord. He shook his head in horror.

I met Joan's eyes and we both smiled, and of course I offered her the scissors – she'd done everything else, done it her way – and she nodded tranquilly, said to her husband, 'Take a picture of this,' and cut the cord herself.

For me, that's the epitome of a woman celebrating her strength. Lots of birthing women cut their own umbilical cords in labours I'm present at – and also in my books. It's something very simple but very powerful, and it makes me smile every time.

I began as a hospital-trained general nurse, as nearly all midwives did before the universities rose to the challenge of increasing the professional standing of midwifery education and assumed the mantle of training midwives in Australia.

Nursing was a growth experience for a girl of seventeen in the late seventies: first full-time job, an eight-hour drive away from rural parents, and living fairly freely in the nurses' home in a capital city. But it wasn't the culture shock of a city that made me grow up; it was the sudden exposure to surgery, illness, accidents and tragedy that happened to real people who were out of their own environment, sick, and in need of my help. As a nurse, my job was to support these patients in their crisis of illness, and the whole focus was to create order out of chaos and wait for the doctor's round so they could be healed.

Nursing is filled with incredible people who teach by

example, and the specialties and medicines involved are diverse and complicated. In the time I was a general nurse, I felt I needed to choose a field of medicine to even touch the edges of the scope of disease and treatment options, and no field resonated with me – until I discovered midwifery.

As a student midwife in 1982, with midwifery training still based in hospitals, this meant going back to being the junior nurse after finally becoming a sister, but to my mind midwifery was more fulfilling, more emotionally demanding, and occasionally more tragic than nursing. This was where I wanted to be.

Even though it was still an era when women were told how to birth by imperfect but powerful doctors, suited men who left cigarettes burning on the windowsills outside labour wards, there were small stirrings of change. Thank goodness for the empathetic doctors who were there for all the right reasons, or I may have had to walk away for my own sanity. How times have changed – in those days husbands weren't encouraged to be present at birth, let alone male or female partners with different surnames, but now it is not uncommon for the supporting parent to be encouraged to lift the newborn baby to the mother's chest.

My husband and I had our first child in the city, with the help of an uninterested midwife and a wonderful doctor, so I realised it wasn't the profession but the people that made the difference. I wanted to be one of those people who made the difference.

When I finally began to practise as a country midwife, I discovered I had the best job in the world. Being a midwife is a passion that has shaped so much of my life.

I started my post-training midwifery career at the small rural hospital I still work at. I was lucky to come in at a changing-of-the-guard time; the older midwives stayed around long enough to share their amazing skills before they retired and we, the next generation of midwives, were all around the same age. So we grew as midwives together, birthed each other's children, grew families, shared schooling dramas and became a close-knit team. Now we're growing grandchildren, and because it's a small town, the mothers of our birthing women tell their daughters about how we were there when they were born.

I was blessed to be a mum five times and those experiences reinforced that each birth is different, that your midwife in labour has a huge impact not just on the way your birth progresses, but even how you see yourself and the job you've just done.

I was also lucky enough to join a not-for-profit group of midwives and doctors who volunteer a weekend several times a year to teach systematic approaches to obstetric emergencies. The added bonus to refreshing my own skills is the chance to meet and network with doctors and midwives from all over Australia. A lot of those midwives appear in this book.

Writing is my second love. The funny thing is, I didn't sell my first fiction book until I wrote about midwives and midwifery and the women we care for. I've written many medical romance novels, heavy on midwifery and light on romance, two self-help birth books, and now this non-fiction collection – a whole new adventure I can't wait to share with you.

When I was asked to write this book, I discovered how many

different types of midwifery there are in the vastness of Australia, and how exciting it was to share just a few of those stories.

This book is a window into different settings of midwifery, which nonetheless all uphold the intrinsic privilege of being a part of the birthing family's experience, and a celebration of the miracles we see every day when midwives go to work.

CHAPTER 2

Grassroots midwifery

Rae Condon

Rae Condon moves quietly through the darkened room. She brings with her an aura of calm, competence, and total belief in the strength of the mother as the labour builds. Rae's voice holds a cadence that somehow dissipates tension, and you see the woman's shoulders droop a little as she releases the muscles she's hitched to try to pull away from the contraction. The mum's breath sighs out, she lifts her head, smiles, and the mood in the room shifts from anxiety to anticipation.

There have been many midwifery settings in Rae's career, as a tertiary hospital midwife, a rural midwife, a sole practitioner in remote area antenatal clinics and a homebirth midwife. At the moment, she's on the east coast of New South Wales working in a large rural hospital. They're lucky to have her. Amid the distraction of a busy hospital, Rae quietly goes about caring for women the way they want to be cared for.

Rae likes a simple lifestyle and lives on a farm with her husband, Brian. He's a gentle soul, clever with his hands, and happy to dive into fun stuff like kayaking, camping and pushbike riding, and even followed his wife through central Australia for an extended working holiday in remote locations.

I laughed when Rae told me that 'nursing didn't float my boat' all those years ago when she was a student nurse – until the day she started her rotation in the midwifery unit and saw her first baby being born. You can hear the magic, the entrancement in her voice as she remembers that first birth. It's funny how a stranger can change your life, isn't it? A woman whose name Rae doesn't remember, whose baby could be a parent to many babies now. That's how being a midwife can affect you.

'I could feel the hormones flowing and I was hooked.' You can't miss the light in Rae's eyes as she says that. And of course she spent the rest of that day boring everyone to death by talking about any and all aspects of the labour or birth. Anything that would keep her reliving the experience. A lot of midwives do that the first time.

She's straight out with it. 'I struggled through becoming a registered nurse only to become eligible to become a midwife.' Nowadays aspiring midwives can go straight into midwifery with a Bachelor of Midwifery (many still do a Bachelor of Nursing first) but Rae trained in the mid seventies at a major teaching hospital.

Terms like 'women-centred' were rare in the seventies.

There were strict, dubious regimes under which mothers were separated from their babies under the guise of 'we know best', and fathers could not accompany the mothers unless they were married and sometimes not even then. For people like Rae it was hard to watch – a theme that reappears throughout this anthology with other midwives and something that encouraged many of them to fight for change.

Rae shakes her head as she remembers as a new student holding a woman's hand, with the midwife – a nun – bellowing for the mother to push, while her partner was outside the door. 'That woman refused to push because he wasn't in the room.' Her face clouds as she adds, 'I regret to this day that I didn't walk over and open the door and invite him in.' She didn't have the confidence then that she has now.

'Some of those midwifery nuns were angels, but others were a fierce bunch,' Rae says with a shake of the head, 'but that hierarchical system filtered down through the other midwives, which left the student midwife in no doubt about their lack of importance within the unit.

'Thank goodness for your mates, all in the same boat, which made the year quite fun – and of course the women made you feel that you had contributed to their birth experience and that made all the difference.' Rae remembers, as a student, holding a birthing woman's hand; when the midwife told Rae to get her gloves on, the woman wouldn't let go of her. Eventually the midwife swapped places and Rae can clearly remember when 'Emily' slid into the world. 'I still have her photo; she'd be about forty now.' Many years on, Rae is still profoundly touched by the women she serves. 'I've never wanted to do anything else.'

In her early years as a registered midwife Rae mostly worked in rural base hospitals. Unfortunately these too were hierarchical, and intervention was often the norm. By 'intervention' Rae means procedures that in 2015 we realise didn't need doing, but were carried out because they 'had always been done'. Things like intravenous cannulas and drips for every woman just in case of disaster, enemas and pubic hair shaves as soon as a woman walked through the door in early labour, and epidurals as the preferred method for pain relief. And birth attendants shouting at women to push. It just didn't feel right. Frustrated, Rae moved on again with Brian.

Eventually Rae began working in a small country hospital that had a birth rate of about a hundred per year. Thankfully, here women were encouraged to use resources like water, heat and massage to manage their labour and birth; women made decisions, communicated their needs and got on with birthing their babies. Rae was in heaven; this caring environment fitted her like a glove.

As a natural progression, she moved into assisting women to birth babies in their own homes in her spare time. Rae shakes her head again and smiles. 'It seemed to me the roles were reversed and these women became the teachers and carers of birth and I once again became the student.'

She had an exercise book in which she detailed all their antenatal care, and at the end of the pregnancy she'd describe their birth journey and then would leave the book with the mothers as a journal. The midwives kept other notes of their own, just like hospital records, but women loved and never lost their journals. Not surprisingly, in the time Rae and her close midwife friend, Kath, ran their little homebirthing service, several women that they cared for shared more than one birth with them.

Sometimes it was a challenge, like the woman who contacted them for her next homebirth and mentioned in passing, 'By the way, I'm having twins.' Rae remembers that she made all sorts of excuses to not be involved – as midwives out on their own it was considered a statistically dangerous venture. 'I took on our obstetric fear regarding her twin pregnancy,' Rae admits. 'Even though I'd been there for her previous birth and knew how centred she was, I let my usual belief in women and birth and human design drift away.'

But that woman must have known they'd be there for her and could be swayed, because Rae can still remember her words – 'I understand,' the woman said with a serene smile. 'But let's see how we go.' No pressure – or was there?

Rae says, 'Whenever I had doubts I just seemed to be surrounded by influential, strong women. My friend Kath and I shared our concerns and joys, then got on with helping women at home.' Many experienced midwives were taking on the system and standing up for what they believed was right and just for birthing women. 'Midwives were starting to recognise that birthing women themselves knew what was needed and that they were fighting to birth their babies their way.'

The family with twins taught Rae amazing lessons about

fear-based decision-making and remembering to support women to have control over their birth experiences. 'It seems to me we are still asking women to trust their bodies to birth babies – and yet we don't trust women to have that ability?'

So what was it like that day when her twin lady went into labour and called them to her home for the birth? Was there trepidation? Excitement?

Remembering it, Rae nods and scrunches up her face to concentrate. She grins and then her face takes on a dreamy look.

'The mother and babies were in perfect harmony. We'd shared lots of antenatal care, they'd grown to a good size at 39 weeks, lined themselves up perfectly, headfirst for birth.'

The labouring woman sat in the corner of the room on a mattress with pillows around her, like a queen with everyone waiting to be there for her. Her husband hovered, quietly attuned to her needs, and their two-year-old son and six-year-old daughter would sidle up to her and lay their cheeks against hers, just for a moment, and she'd hug them gently and, reassured, the children would drift off again. Her best friend was there, offering her pieces of fruit or water, and her friend's husband waited quietly in the background with their four-year-old boy and the other children.

There was so much food. It was celebration, this birth. People would offer the mother little morsels and everyone else grazed. Everyone had been preparing for days for this feast.

And the mother had been preparing for nine months. It was a serene, two-hour labour, Rae or Kath leaning in with their little portable Dopplers to amplify the babies' heartbeats so everyone in the room could hear them. And then it was time.

While the mother was pushing in second stage, the young daughter reached out with one small finger and gently touched the crowning head of the baby, amazed as the little thatch of dark hair inched forward to the outside world. Her brother copied her, creeping forward to touch the baby's hair, then dodged back. This was the family birth the mother wanted, and as the first fellow birthed there was a sigh of joy throughout the room.

Rae says, 'They were both headfirst. We broke her waters after the first twin, and the next boy followed shortly after.'

There was a blow-up child's pool, waist deep, in the room, filled with warm water. They didn't use it for labour; they used it after the birth, when the mother, father, babies and their two siblings climbed in to share a family bath. It was what the mother wanted, and was not something that would have happened in a hospital birth.

Today, Rae runs private birth and parenthood preparation classes, and is strongly committed to women being well-prepared for labour and birth and feeling confident with their partner offering the support they need. She believes in the importance of the couple developing a positive mindset so the fear factor doesn't interfere with the hormonal flow. She wants couples to retain control over the decision-making process during their birth experience, and not to be coerced into intervention they may regret later.

One of Rae's couples remembers her saying, 'Fear equals tension equals pain. You must breathe.'

Rae says that while her general nursing years were drudgery and she often wanted to quit, midwifery is a joy that grows more satisfying the longer she is a midwife.

Her face clouds. 'However, I have never felt comfortable with a parent's grief; the lost baby that stopped growing for whatever reason. It's so overwhelming, sad and mostly unfair.' The reality of birth is that it's not always a happy, euphoric event. Sometimes babies die, a part of the parents die, midwives and doctors grieve for the potential snatched away, and everyone involved is left forever wondering what they could have done differently.

One such time, in a very small rural hospital, a place of thirty or so births a year, Rae was called to a birth as a second midwife. When the little girl was born, she didn't breathe, and eventually the desperate resuscitation measures had to stop. 'I think that is the hardest way – expectation builds, everything goes forward normally, and then a baby arrives who for some reason can't live without her mother exchanging oxygen for her. Thank goodness it doesn't happen often, but it happens.' The other midwife at this birth was very young, and became distraught and soon went home. As the only midwife, Rae was left to deal with shocked, grieving parents she barely knew. She still worries that she must have appeared distant and aloof as she went about the tasks that had still to be completed before she could let the walls crumble and allow herself to grieve.

But there are happy times too. Partners react differently to the birth of their children; most men have tears in their eyes or streaming down their faces, some sob unreservedly with relief and joy. One partner, Rae remembers, abruptly left the room as the baby was born. The staff exchanged glances at his strange behaviour, then heard an enormous clattering crash just outside the room as he fainted, knocking over a trolley of equipment. Nearly everyone ran out, leaving the mother and baby still looking at each other. Another young man was so ecstatic he grabbed each person in the room in turn and hugged them, lifting Rae off her feet in disregard of the sterile field, and twirling her around and before moving on to the next person. His elation filled the room with a release of laughter and merriment.

At the moment, Rae works in a large rural hospital where she experiences some magic moments but a little too much intervention, and feels she may have to find somewhere with more women-centred care.

Today is a typical day in the busy area, which consists of four birth rooms and two beds for outpatient assessment. There are two midwives in birthing; their shift starts at 7 a.m. and they go off at 3.30 p.m. This is what they pack into their day.

In Room 1, Serene Sarah is in established labour at about 6 centimetres (two-thirds of the way). She has been labouring all night, but is determined to birth this baby in her own time, declining an offer by the on-call doctor to try to hurry the labour. Her partner and mother are with her, doing the major job of support, and Rae discreetly drifts in and out until she is needed; there's so much more for her to attend to in the other rooms.

In Room 2 there sits a tense, non-English-speaking woman and her husband who have stayed overnight because they refused to go home; the mother has had contractions that seemed to stop and start (a sign that she is still early in labour and it may even stop again), but they're too worried the baby will come to feel safe at home. They sit wringing their hands, burning eyes latching onto Rae as she sits with them. With a little to and fro from the interpreter and some discussion, the woman, reassured, eventually consents to go home to encourage the arrival of her regular contractions in the more peaceful environment away from a busy labour ward.

In another room, a young woman with red hair is admitted for induction at 41 weeks and 4 days. Her heavily tattooed boyfriend is disappointed when the doctor says the baby won't come soon. 'Can't you make it come quicker?'

Rae explains that Prostin gel is used to soften the opening of the cervix and trigger hormones that will bring on labour; meanwhile, the young woman will be transferred back to the ward to await either labour or further applications of gel, and their baby may not arrive today.

Before Rae can return to Serene Sarah, a first-time mother is admitted for assessment, having ruptured her membranes three days prior. It is decided to induce labour because of the risk of infection. The mum is pleased with this decision, as her leaking of fluid has been worrying her, and she was quite distressed when she arrived. The student midwife is available to assist with her care, which allows Rae to check on another admission.

Now another first-time mother is admitted in early labour at 40 weeks and 2 days. The couple have attended hypno-birthing classes, and have support people and a doula with them. They have brought a very descriptive birth plan with highlighted points, such as having a water birth, the partner birthing the baby, and a physiological third stage (no injection to hasten the birth of the placenta – so waiting up to an hour for the natural expulsion of the placenta from the mother's body). After a preliminary assessment this woman declines a vaginal assessment. The glide of Rae's hands over the wom-an's belly tells her it is likely the baby is posterior and needs to rotate. This will take time, movement and good contractions, and it is unlikely she will birth before Rae goes home.

Lunchtime has come and gone. The desk phone rings con-stantly; diet aide, ward staff, general practice doctors and women seeking advice makes for constant noise and neces-sitates good time-management skills. In this typical day in a busy hospital, Rae is spread too thinly to hear each woman's needs or concerns, which is frustrating because she's not giv-ing the care she would if she had the time. It makes her long to go back to homebirthing, with the woman's faith in herself and choice the major factors.

Serene Sarah is getting closer now, but Rae has time for one more assessment before she settles in the birth room.

A woman at 32 weeks' gestation presents very distressed because she's taken her blood pressure and found it concerning.

After a cardiotocograph (CTG) assessment, which measures the rate and variation of the baby's heartbeat, particularly during the presence of any contractions or tightenings, and several checks of the woman's blood pressure, she is discharged home with advice on warning signs and suggestions on re-presenting to the ward if concerns arise.

Now the red-headed woman's boyfriend is upset because the next dose of Prostin gel has been delayed until a birth room becomes available. Rae needs to take time to reassure him that the induction will go ahead as soon as possible.

Rae steps away from the mayhem and settles in the corner of Sarah's bathroom to wait. The room is quiet, the light dim, the cacophony outside seems a distant dream, and before long, Sarah quietly births a baby girl in the big white bath. Mother and baby are snuggled together, skin to skin, still in the birth room when Rae goes home, thankful for a peaceful birth to end the day.

However, all days are different. Her next shift has a lull, with just one couple to care for, and the midwifery angels are smiling because she's met them a few years ago at one of her Calmbirth classes. This woman is loved and supported; she knows her own strength, and she knows how to birth her babies. In fact, she loves birthing babies. After many deeply considered conversations with her husband, and meetings with all concerned, her pregnancy and coming birth are a precious gift as a surrogate arrangement for a same-sex couple.

This baby is small, much smaller than her previous babies, and as she is term, the obstetric experts encourage an induction to hasten the birth and avoid compromising the baby's wellbeing. The woman is not convinced there is potential risk; she argues the different genetic material has produced a smaller baby, and the baby's movements are reassuring to her. However, she feels the weight of the surrogate parents' concern for the baby's wellbeing, as they too have listened to the obstetric argument. The woman capitulates and the induction commences.

Labour is slow to start, then builds in momentum. The intending parents give the woman, who is supported by her husband, lots of privacy while still being a part of their child's birth. The woman is very generous, talking with them and reassuring them while getting on with birthing this baby.

As the energy builds the woman sinks into a warm, deep bath, though the obstetrician has requested she births out of the water at the end in case the small baby becomes distressed. The light is dim and she is cradled by her husband as his soothing words wash over her; they spend this time alone. Rae watches quietly from the corner, soaking in the magic yet watchful. Then everything speeds up: the woman feels an urge to push and the baby's head is born as the woman is asked to birth out of the bath. She agrees and positions herself on hands and knees with her head resting in her husband's lap. The intending parents are invited to witness their child's arrival, and Rae guides one new parent's hands to cup and support the baby's head as the body eases out. The newborn is gathered into anxious hands; a small baby girl, beautiful, healthy and lusty, letting everyone know she has birthed. The atmosphere is charged with disbelieving emotion, and tears, laughing, kissing, gratitude and baby noise fill the room. Rae savours the experience.

This is her space. Part of the environment and atmosphere, in a privileged place, she is able to share the euphoria and joy of a baby moving from the internal to the external world. How many people have jobs like that?

CHAPTER 3

The negotiator and breech

Kate Braye

The mother sits on a birth stool, leaning back into her husband's chest. The stool is open at the front, and the baby's bottom can be seen inching out. They are in a hospital room with six people in attendance, but nobody speaks or touches the baby. The sound of the woman's slow breathing mixes with the *clop*, *clop*, *clop* of the baby's heartbeat from the sensor strapped around her belly. Within a minute the umbilical cord slithers down with the abdomen, and the baby's legs pull up and jiggle, almost as if pedalling a pushbike. Still no interfering hands interrupt the weight of the baby as it shifts itself down the birth passage. The armpits appear, and chubby arms sweep the chest as the shoulders turn and birth. A few seconds later, drawn by gravity, the baby's chin and face appear and it is done. The midwife gathers and the mother's hands reach to lift her baby against her breasts.

When the baby cries, the birthing mother grins and gives a victory salute. She's birthed this baby who came bottom first without a caesarean – a decision many women would not have had the option of choosing – because this was the way she wanted to birth her baby.

Kate Braye, the woman's midwife, strongly believes that babies directly benefit from the tenacity of their mothers. Kate loves watching babies come bottom first, even though she knows that in this obstetric climate it is less stressful for Mum when they turn to come headfirst, because the art and science of natural, safe breech birth is only just re-emerging thanks to the support of a growing number of midwives like Kate, and obstetricians like Dr Andrew Bisits, all over the world.

Kate is calmly proper, with a slight English accent, but has an unexpected laugh that makes you smile back. As a facilitator helping someone to gain confidence in a new skill, she's not just teaching, she's invested and excited when your learning happens. Kate's biggest strengths are her love of acquiring knowledge for evidence-based reasoning, and in being a quietly resourceful negotiator for birthing women who want to make their own decision about mode of birth.

Kate works in a tertiary hospital and as a private midwife in women's homes. 'Women don't sign up for my idea of their birth experience; this is their adventure, so I want to hear their plan and help them achieve it.' Kate's there whether women birth in their home or hospital, and they can make up their minds about their options at the last minute before their due date.

Kate believes that before a woman is pregnant it's possible – probable, really – that she doesn't have any formed intention about the place and manner in which she will birth her first child. Yet, when she is about to birth, and even more so if she has limitations on her choices, the way she births can be one of the most important occasions of her life. The way she is listened to in her birth planning is the cornerstone of her mothering platform – her self-esteem as a mother that she draws from in the years ahead – and she needs to have her say and be heard. Kate is the negotiator when a mother is most vulnerable, for example being told her baby is breech late in pregnancy and being pressured into an automatic caesarean birth without discussion.

So how did Kate become a midwife? Despite an early love of learning, Kate grew up in England in a time when girls left school at sixteen and were found a job.

She worked quite happily for the Inland Revenue, but across town the hospital beckoned, and at eighteen she was accepted to train as a nurse. Kate loved nursing, and was so proud of her profession she marched around the hospital in her uniform glowing with pride. She enjoyed every part of it, and remembers with a twinkle in her eye the absolute joy of the gorgeous red sash she was permitted to wear in her second year.

It was in this hospital that Kate met and fell in love with her handsome Australian doctor. Three years later she finished her general training, and after six months' postgraduate experience decided midwifery would be a useful addition to her skills and was able to train in England before she left for Australia.

Kate found such joy in the eighteen months of birthing babies in the relaxed environment of a woman's own home with the Home Midwifery Service, that she was sad to leave. When she moved to Australia and back into the midwifery workforce, the care of labouring women was much different from that in England.

After Kate and her husband settled in Australia, and after the birth of their own babies – three natural births – Kate went back to midwifery, but even then she knew the key to greater job satisfaction was her own education.

In Australia she felt she was more of a 'nurse to the obstetricians' than a midwife to the women. The doctors were all-powerful and usually backed by indoctrinated midwives well-versed in medical intervention. Kate joined the underground movement of quietly rebellious midwives who became experts at protecting women from often less-than-sensitive interventions.

With a judiciously timed phone call Kate could delay a doctor's arrival to allow him or her no time to intervene in the natural process; she could save a perineum by misplacing the episiotomy scissors; she could suggest the woman was not quite ready to push to allow her extra time to achieve an unassisted birth. Thankfully times have changed, women and midwives have found their voices and choices are now there to be made about birth time, mode and interventions.

Over the next few years Kate worked part-time, was a

mother and wife, and took numerous courses to appease her thirst for knowledge. She trained as a child and family health nurse to learn more about the first years of a child's life so she could help the families she worked with. When that was done she studied for her Sexual Health Diploma to extend her knowledge of contraception and sexual health and then went on to become a lactation consultant to increase her toolbox of resources for breastfeeding mothers. Still driven to learn, this busy young mum commenced her Masters in Midwifery, though in the difficulties that followed her studies had moments of surrealism – more a blur than a memory.

Study fragmented when family tragedy struck. Kate's mum, in England, became terminally ill and Kate flew back and forth between two continents. Then Kate's daughter was diagnosed with cancer at ten years of age, and Kate spent another heart-breaking year studying on and off at her daughter's bedside in the hospital until the little girl won her courageous battle for recovery.

More study followed, and then more disaster when Kate's daughter, now fifteen, suffered a relapse and her cancer came back with a vengeance.

Again Kate was typing assignments beside a hospital bed, this time to stay sane despite the worry and fear for her family. Kate's daughter fought her way to wellness again, and suddenly the Masters in Midwifery was done.

Kate remembers the poignancy when her father flew out from England, bursting with pride to see his daughter, the first of any of their family to graduate from university with such honour, and the family smiled again.

Kate acknowledges that her daughter's ill health had a positive impact on how she saw the sacred value of all her family's lives, influenced what she did with her own life, and gave her valuable insight into the fear of loss in a birth crisis with the women she cared for. 'Life and death in birth is such a rollercoaster. I want to be there on tragic occasions as well as joyful ones, to nurture and help grieving families create memories and find themselves as parents in that very brief window of time before their child leaves them.'

As one of the original midwives at the John Hunter Hospital Team Midwifery Service in the early 1990s, a time when one midwife (with a buddy midwife as back-up) caring for a woman throughout her pregnancy was rare in Australia, Kate spent four years in innovative collaboration with the doctors to provide women-centred care. Since then, team midwifery has stayed close to Kate's heart.

It was here she met Dr Andrew Bisits, an obstetrician and advocate for women's right to choose vaginal breech birth, in spite of the prevailing climate of fear and misconceptions about breech birth, and Kate supported women in considering that option.

'Some doctors don't talk about the increased risk of special care nursery admission for caesarean babies. They don't mention the impact of a surgical birth on future pregnancies. Vaginal breech birth should be an option that's discussed and if baby, mother and birthplace/carers are aligned can be the safest option in the long term.'

Years later Kate went on to be one of the core team of midwives and doctors spreading this message and refreshing breech delivery skills in the BABE (Becoming a Breech Expert) course, with Dr Bisits. These courses seek to share the knowledge and revitalise declining breech-birthing skills among doctors and midwives all over Australia.

Back in 2007 at Belmont Birth Centre, a standalone birth centre in Newcastle, NSW, Kate found the home in midwifery she'd been seeking. Belmont offered women undisturbed birth: birthing in the way they wanted, sometimes outside the square of expected care, their choice supported by a mantle of safety – a considered awareness of risk and a plan in place if escalation to a higher level of care should be needed – but with the provision of options, such as homebirth or birth centre birth away from a hospital – enabling the undisturbed birth they otherwise wouldn't have. Kate believes she could have gone through her whole career without experiencing such fulfilment in her work as she did at Belmont, and she is truly thankful for her time there.

Now that she is working in private practice, sometimes risk factors in pregnancy do fall outside the boundaries of low risk that Kate and her midwifery partner work within if birthing at home. In this event, Kate works to stem the way decisions begin to slide out of the mother's hands when something unexpected crops up and they need to birth in the hospital environment. She remembers one such occasion well.

Michelle, at 37 weeks, was suddenly confronted with a baby that was breech, and shuddered at the thought of having a caesarean birth. Despite trying all the natural methods as well as her obstetrician attempting to change the baby's position, Michelle's baby remained bottom first. So Kate couldn't promise the undisturbed vaginal birth Michelle wanted, but they could direct their energies towards achievable goals. Kate negotiated for allowing natural labour time at home before admission to the hospital for intense monitoring, to make sure the labour started with the right energy.

Kate was aware that in hospital there would probably be no labouring in the bath due to continuous monitoring, maybe even lying on the bed instead of sitting up as Michelle preferred. It depended on the doctor rostered on for that time and how comfortable that obstetrician was with vaginal breech birth.

When Michelle's labour started, Kate remembers, 'I came around the side of their house and saw Michelle holding on to a thick twisted rope, so she could reach up on the rope when the contractions came, with Adrian doing soft-touch massage on her back. They were outside under an awning overhang – rain sheeting down in front of her nose, not wetting her, the air electrically charged.

'It was brilliant,' Kate says. 'They looked so beautiful. Adrian leaning over her protectively, the attitude of their bodies, the surrendering, letting the hormones do their thing. It was perfect.

'I didn't interrupt. Early first stage of labour is an important time for mothers to allow their bodies to ease into the work ahead. Early contractions can be "scared away" if you pay too much mind to them. I left them and went inside and waited until they called me. They knew I was there. Women in labour feel so much more comfortable with a clinician known to them, and I feel privileged that women are comfortable with me. Truly, it's a great thing, and demonstrating that is so satisfying to share with students. When that light bulb goes on for a student, it can change their career.

'When I came out again Michelle was well established in labour, there would be no stopping it now, and we drove to the hospital.' Michelle's labour had definitely started with the right energy.

Kate dropped them at the entrance of the hospital and parked her car. Upstairs they were blessed with a very forward-thinking doctor, a man who trusted Kate and believed in safe vaginal breech birth. For Michelle, everything was calm again. All discussions or negotiations were carried on outside the door, because negotiations were Kate's job, not Michelle's. 'She had her own job to do. Michelle didn't need to move from birthing brain to negotiation brain.'

Kate was the person in charge of the safety issues, and listened to the baby carefully, watched Michelle's progress, and negotiated for her to use the positions she wanted instead of the bed as the labour progressed.

It was all going really well, then contrarily, for no reason, the contractions went away. The baby's heart rate slowed, and Kate asked Michelle to push.

'Okay, Michelle. We need your baby now.' Responding to the calm emphasis in the midwife she trusted, Michelle pushed even harder, and then it was done.

Max, who did come breech, was stunned from the birth, but babies are so responsive to stimulation that within ten minutes he was back to his mother's chest healthy and crying.

Michelle's mood switched from utter determination to pure elation that she had the experience she had. So many women aren't given the same opportunity, but are just told 'breech presentation: no discussion, caesarean section booked'. That's why Kate loves what she does.

'All this research backs women knowing what they need to do. It's so bad for the women's health, including mental health, to have the decision taken away from them. To be told their instinct is wrong to want to birth a breech. For Michelle, this was the best thing she could do in that environment.'

But immersion in other people's pregnancies and births does require sacrifice. After seven years of being on call almost all the time for birthing women, sharing homebirths and birth centre births and extreme joy and sadness, it was time for a break.

Kate's father became terminally ill in the UK, and after he died Kate did what she always did in a crisis: she studied. Kate returned to university and started a PhD.

The academic workload was her heaviest yet, and unable to secure a part-time role in caseload midwifery, Kate reluctantly left Belmont Birth Centre and returned part-time to the tertiary hospital in Newcastle. But it's turned out to be a good thing. With her strength in advocacy, Kate hopes to introduce more autonomy for midwives and in that way increase the women-centred care for birthing women in the large and busy teaching hospital.

Currently she works four days a fortnight in the hospital, is in the second year of her PhD, and is a partner in a private midwifery practice. Sometimes when she suggests homebirth, the fathers pale, but she's very supportive of their reaction: 'It's the guy's job to think of safety, so they go through the whole homebirth discussion.'

As well, Kate teaches ALSO (Advanced Life Support in Obstetrics), on a volunteer basis, with and to like-minded doctors and midwives from all over Australia, and the BABE course.

Now, on the days that she works with Dan, her midwifery colleague, Kate is in a good space. Homebirth requires a high level of commitment to study as well as a commitment to be available almost twenty-four seven for women and their families. There are births in women's homes at odd hours, and Kate is a registered immuniser, has advanced neonatal resuscitation skills, is medically endorsed to order medications like antibiotics and vitamin K, and ready to deal with obstetric emergencies if they crop up. If needed, she can initiate treatment and arrange transport of women to a higher level of care.

Then there are busy shifts in the hospital, where Kate negotiates outside the room for the woman inside. There is volunteer teaching on weekends in different cities in Australia, the opportunity to learn from other professionals, and a PhD to work on.

What do midwives like Kate, married with children and

family crises and the real world of long hours and full commitment, receive in return for being there so fully for other women? 'Sometimes advocating for women can seem a struggle, but aim to get moments of what a mother needs, and often you'll get all that she needs.' Kate's quiet voice fills with conviction. 'Be the advocate for her. Doing what I do is a privilege and a joy, and I can't imagine doing anything else.'

CHAPTER 4

Small-town midwife

Lisa Ferguson

Lisa Ferguson believes midwives are a lot like swans. Swans glide over the water, serene and majestic, but underneath they are constantly paddling. Midwives look cool on the outside, but underneath, paddling beneath the surface, they are always on the alert for the needs of the birthing woman.

Lisa lives in Temora, a small town in the northern Riverina area of New South Wales, eighty kilometres from Wagga Wagga and two hours from Canberra. Temora, richly agricultural and steeped in gold-rush history, has a population of about 4500 people and smaller-town midwifery is the setting of her story.

Lisa finished her nurses' training in 1979 and her midwifery in 1981, in Sydney. Her midwifery training flew by and she stayed for a year after graduation at the Liverpool

Hospital to consolidate her new skills, and then went to the Royal Hospital in Brisbane to gain more experience.

On a holiday break in New Zealand she met and fell in love with an Australian farmer from Temora, where eventually they settled into their new life together. Away from the city Lisa had to learn to be a country wife and mother, and because midwifery jobs were hard to come by – Temora had about 120 births a year, and nearby Harden and Gundagai about 20–30 births a year – she practised her midwifery in several country hospitals. In her late thirties Lisa added to her workload by teaching antenatal classes in Cootamundra.

Lisa especially loved her time in Cootamundra, a slightly bigger town of 5500 people, the birthplace of Donald Bradman, and the home of the Coota Beach Volleyball Competition – how Australian is that! – a yearly event in which truckloads of sand are carted into the main street to create a fake Kuta Beach. You can tell this country town has a great sense of humour!

Lisa admired the amazing midwives at Cootamundra Hospital who became her role models, and by watching them she saw her own midwifery skills grow. Lisa remembers a wonderful GP who was a progressive forward thinker and gave so much to the community, and he was a stickler for patient welfare, so safety was never compromised in their tiny hospital with few resources. This was the time she looked at the role of the midwife in helping women to find relaxation tools other than medical pain relief. No epidurals were available because of the lack of anaesthetists and yet the women managed beautifully with natural methods of staying calm in labour. These women went from the bath to the birth ball, rocking back and forth, then to the shower and back again until delivery – there wasn't any other choice. It was here that Lisa really honed her skills not just as a midwife but in being with a woman during her labour and birth and knowing how to help that woman in the moment.

Lisa is a strong supporter of the belief that women can understand and accept the way in which the uterus functions naturally during childbirth when free of fear, believing in and trusting their body to do its job. Lisa says, 'If your body knows how to conceive a pregnancy, adapt to all the hormonal and physical changes, grow a fetus and get to term, then it knows how to birth a baby.' When Lisa began to study and share her faith in hypnobirthing, she saw the benefits in the birthing room, and has shared those tools of self-reliance in her care of women.

'You trust your body to function for you every day; you don't tell your heart to beat or your kidneys to work, your body just does it. It can be the same for labour and birthing. Stay relaxed and in a positive mindset, listening to your body and doing what it tells you to do, and your birth can be a very empowering moment in your life.'

Lisa's hypnobirthing classes, and the practice the women did at home listening to the recorded sessions, reminded mothers and support people about the ill-effects of the fear-tension-pain cycle on the birthing process and were some-thing new in a country town. Lisa also shared skills such as visualisation, meditation and relaxation that encourage the body to birth faster and with more comfort by using the learnt prompts during labour when those tendrils of fear crept in.

The first baby Lisa met as a birthing midwife is etched in her memory because first babies for midwives do that. This baby was named Ellie, a beautiful name, and Lisa remembers the mother telling her she was named after a character in the TV show *Dallas*. The thought still makes her smile. The wonder of being at Ellie's birth changed her world forever. Ellie became a special name for Lisa because it reoccurred several times during her career. Perhaps the most impactful Ellie was the beautiful baby of a sixteen-year-old girl whom Lisa met and had the privilege to assist in birth. Like other young women in their teens who find themselves pregnant, Sissy had to make decisions that would affect her for the rest of her life and Lisa was in awe of her composure. Lisa knew that in life, a teen mum without resources faces tough choices: to watch and feel her baby grow then consider giving him or her up for adoption at birth, or accept the stigma and social disadvantages of being a very young mum and perhaps not be able to return to school while caring for her child, or even to terminate the pregnancy and forever wonder what that child would have been like. Unlike less fortunate girls, Sissy had great support in the form of her mother and both her grandmothers, and Lisa remembers how heartwarming it was to see how united families could be in this situation in an era when stigma was prevalent.

The family had listened to Sissy discuss her options and

encouraged her to work through each decision in her own time. Sissy had finally chosen to continue the pregnancy and give her baby up for adoption, but in the last month or so found that she couldn't part with her child.

Supporting her decision, Sissy's mother and grandmothers had made a pact to help the young mum and baby in turns to allow Sissy to have the baby but also still go to school and be a normal teenager. They said that of course they had plenty of time and love that they could give to this child.

When the time came for the birthing room, Lisa remembers these three strong older women took it in turns to guide Sissy through her labour, keeping her focused and relaxed, their sole purpose to just be there for her. As the midwife, Lisa says her job was a joy – monitor the baby and the mother's labour progress, and sit quietly back and savour the strength in the room.

When the baby was born, Sissy named her Ellie Rose. Ellie's name means 'light', and she always shone as special for Lisa.

Lisa remembers saying to the male doctor who had attended the birth that he looked out of place amid all the woman power in the room – four generations of women and a female midwife – and he had smilingly agreed. When she received a card and flowers from the family thanking her several weeks later she remembers it as a humbling experience.

Lisa didn't see Sissy again until she presented in labour several years later. At first they didn't remember each other from Sissy's first birth, but why would they? At sixteen Sissy had had the support of people much more significant to her than her midwife. And Lisa only recognised her after they began discussing Sissy's other children and Sissy mentioned her first daughter, Ellie Rose.

Lisa considers it the greatest privilege to have been present for the birth of Sissy's third child because she'd never forgotten Ellie's birth. Sissy had finished school, this was her third child with Ellie Rose's father, and she was a strong woman in her own right with a beautiful family after such a stressful time at the beginning. Smaller-town midwifery is like that, with your own career growing with families, lives touching and then baby going home, until that family comes back again and you can be a part of their next child's birth.

For Lisa, the hardest part is when she doesn't recognise a woman she's cared for several months after their pregnancies, because they will have changed from when she last saw them, flushed and tired but thrilled with the achievement of birthing their baby. She always feels guilty about that. They'll have since lost all that fluid and changed their hairstyle and will be looking fantastic and totally different. She wishes she could remember them all, because on the day they birthed and she was looking after them, they were the most important people for her – a midwife comes across hundreds of women in the course of their career – and she admires them all.

Lisa now works as the midwifery educator between Temora and other small local hospitals and shares her passion for being with women in birth with new midwives and students.

CHAPTER 5

First-year midwife

Bronwyn Thomas

Broni Thomas is our cover girl and the photo of her and baby Theo Storey, whose mum was cared for postnatally by Broni, was taken by another woman who was supported by Broni in labour. Broni's a country-town girl too, twenty-three, mischievous, and likes to go a little wild on a Friday night – but she can also hold an oxygen mask the size of a fifty-cent piece steady on a tiny premature baby's nose and mouth until specialist help arrives, even if it takes six hours. Broni is a shining example of the new breed of midwife being trained through our universities. She completed her Bachelor of Midwifery degree in 2013, attending her practical placements in a large tertiary hospital.

Broni is bright-eyed and vivacious with genuine people skills developed during her time helping in a baby club at the local chemist. When a woman or visitor walks onto the ward, Broni's smile and welcome is like a warm hug, and you can see the instinctive smile in return from the newcomer. These are the midwives a maternity unit needs to begin that journey of trust around birth.

As a teenager, the last thing Broni expected to do was come back to her small country town to work or settle down. She had dreams she didn't think she would be able to fulfil staying in town. Moving three hours' drive down the highway to Newcastle to study midwifery for three years was the right decision, but love brought her back home when those three years were up. Suddenly she was ecstatic to be starting as a newly graduated midwife at the local hospital. Who would have thought?

Dressed in her new uniform, hair in a long brown ponytail, on her first proper day on the job she was keen to get started and learn new things in a different environment. The ward had an elective caesarean section booked for the day, which was certainly one way to dive into things and Broni bubbled with excitement until she saw the name. It was a girlfriend's sister-in-law, a woman who had always been open about the fact that she wasn't a fan, and Broni knew she wouldn't agree to her being present for the birth. So, returning home to work also meant a welcome back to small-town politics, and she spent her first few days as a registered midwife trying to avoid the ward's only patient.

She must have wondered if this would be a repeat occurrence. 'To be honest, I was embarrassed to even say to the

senior midwives, "I can't look after her, she doesn't like me."
I felt so immature and unprofessional. I realised this was one
of the downsides to coming back to work in a rural town I
went to school in, especially in a profession that is so personal
and special in families' lives.'

Broni started her degree in 2010 and found the first semester of second year at university the toughest to get through.
The study was harder than first year and she was still getting
used to the concept of being on call for the continuity women.
Student midwives closely follow the pregnancies of at least ten
women per year and these women generously agree to allow
the student midwife to share their birth journey. This is how
a fledgling midwife can learn about an individual woman's
needs as opposed to learning about the health system's ideas of
a woman's needs. It also means giving out her personal mobile
phone number for any worries the mum might want to ask her
about, no wild Friday nights in case a mum goes into labour
and she needs to be at the hospital for the birth, and sitting
in on antenatal visits whenever any of the mums has a visit
scheduled at the hospital.

The long-term goal of the Australian College of Midwives
is for every woman in Australia, regardless of where she lives,
to have the option of continuity of care (one midwife – or a
small team of midwives who care for a woman from start to
finish), and it is the framework student midwives learn from in
the universities.

For Broni there were moments when she wondered if midwifery was for her. It took her about half a semester to realise

that her university experience would be different from that of her roommates. The coursework for midwifery required being on call almost twenty-four seven, plus her two part-time jobs meant she was always busy between university, placement, work and maintaining a long-distance relationship. It all seemed too much and too hard, she missed home, and nurturing close relationships with women who were mostly older than her called for a confidence she wasn't sure she had.

'The great thing was,' Broni says, 'one good birth later, and my head was back in the right space.'

Of the forty-five women who started their midwifery degree with Broni, there were only five like her without children. At the time, she thought this put her at a huge disadvantage. Everyone who had kids had so many stories and personal views on the subjects they were learning about, whereas she hadn't heard of any of them. As time went on she came to realise that being childless was more of a blessing than a curse for her. She was a blank slate – everything she learnt at university she learnt with an open unbiased mind.

Broni admired the student mothers trying their hardest to keep up while raising little ones at home and remembers endless tutorials that ended with everyone in tears, talking about how hard it was to leave their babies when called away to a birth. These tutorials made her snap out of any self pity; even though she had her own challenges going on, she decided she had it easy compared to those mums. 'In a way I guess their struggle made me stronger and work harder because I had it easy compared to them.'

In the final semester of her degree she found a new motivation that she hadn't felt before. It may have just been because she was so close to finishing and wanted it to be over, but she found herself impatient to go in to placement every day. She loved being with pregnant women and at last felt competent and confident in her abilities as a midwife. Other midwives around her began to notice and let her take charge. Suddenly Broni wasn't scared as she'd been in her previous placements. She felt ready to become a registered midwife and eager to take responsibility.

She believes she owes so much to the continuity-of-care women who allowed her to share their births during her training. 'It is because of all of those women who allowed me to share their pregnancy journeys that I'm the midwife I am today. Honestly, they were all amazing.' Broni loves continuity of care and believes being able to follow women throughout their pregnancies allows for established relationships of trust and respect prior to labour. This can help support women and babies and prevent feelings of isolation when a woman goes into labour.

Broni remains a little self-conscious about her age and lack of experience. She still finds herself wincing at 'you look too young to be a midwife', which she brushed off the first few times but admits did start to get to her. Thankfully the first pregnant woman she met on her first day of placement was so easygoing and laid-back that she asked Broni if she would like to be at her birth, instead of Broni having to ask her. It was experiences like this that helped Broni ease into learning to be 'with women'. Broni admits her shyness and communication skills needed work because the only real conversations she'd held with women older than herself had been with her mother and her parents' friends.

With continuity of care, she was able to build rapport, develop her communication skills and grow as a person. 'I owe a great deal to these women, they opened up to me and allowed me to be there through such a vulnerable time in their lives. I will always be grateful for that.'

Broni vividly remembers one of her follow-through women who birthed early in the second year of her degree. The woman was having her second baby and they'd built a great rapport throughout her pregnancy. Broni happened to already be at the hospital on this particular day with another of her continuity-of-care women who was being induced when this mother called, sounding anxious and in discomfort, with her labour all happening very fast.

When Broni saw the woman sitting in a wheelchair at the desk moaning in distress, instinctively she came up beside her and placed a hand on her shoulder, said her name and told her she was there. The woman's shoulders automatically relaxed and 'she calmed'. That is still a magic moment for Broni, when she first saw continuity of care working and knew her familiar presence could be of benefit to women. This mother delivered very quickly and Broni remembers how happy she felt to be there with her at the beautiful birth. This was why she wanted to be a midwife.

As a student doing placement in a large city hospital Broni

had the opportunity to work with a large number of midwives in different clinical settings. Here she could discover her pre-ferred areas of care, her own style and where it fitted best, and her niche as a midwife. Some midwives seemed very moth-ering, and Broni was very conscious of the fact that she was young and didn't have any children yet; she feared that women would judge her and wonder if she was capable of providing them with the best care.

Throughout training and during her first year as a regis-tered midwife she learnt to gauge the needs of different women and support their own styles of birth. Some women prefer constant supervision, to be encouraged and sometimes even nudged forward. Other women are happier if she sits silently in the corner and just supports them by her presence. She knows this can change in an instant; something that felt good five minutes ago, can be irritating in this moment – something dads-to-be find out all the time in labour. 'It's not about me. Being "with women" is the most important thing.'

In the small hospital where she now practises full-time, Broni's favourite part is being able to keep track of almost every pregnancy. She loves that someone needs only to say a woman's name and the whole team of midwives already knows their story and when they are due. Broni believes it's so much more personal, allowing for a great environment for women to have their babies in.

Considering four weeks was the longest block of placement she'd completed at university, full-time shiftwork load was a big step up and took a lot of getting used to. In fact, Broni thinks she's still getting used to it. 'I love my sleep – morning shifts are a struggle for me. But once I get to work, it's exciting seeing what is happening in the ward today. Will we have one labour, or two? Or a full postnatal ward? Or maybe only a few postnatal women who we can work closely one-on-one with.'

Broni's local hospital has about 300 births a year which are mostly low risk. Her cousin, a midwife who works in the city, laughs, and mentions her hospital has over 4000 births a year. For Broni, days are very quiet or very busy; there isn't much in between. She thinks that days where she only has one patient can be the most rewarding – when she's able to sit down, have a chat, work through every breastfeed and build a rapport so she can go home feeling like she's had a good day and been helpful.

Not long ago she looked after a woman she knew through mutual friends, who went ahead and had a lovely normal delivery and seemed very pleased with the care provided throughout her labour. However, talking to this mother weeks afterwards Broni was surprised to learn the woman had been thinking that Broni was too inexperienced, and she had initially wanted one of the more senior midwives to look after her. Broni had had no idea of this at the time and felt a little hurt to begin with, but the woman went on to say how happy she was after the fact and that she would recommend Broni to anyone as a midwife during labour. 'Would she have thought that if she hadn't watched me grow up? I guess age will fix that problem.'

Being young and a local, Broni knows many people in the town, and a lot of women her age are having babies. Apart from the student midwives who do placement there, continuity of care with registered midwives isn't available for women in her hospital yet, so she never knows who she will look after. Now, if she finds someone she knows in labour, she asks if it is okay with them if she looks after them.

'I'm not a terrible person so it doesn't happen often that they say yes, but I also believe I have matured a lot in the past eighteen months I've been here. Birth is a woman's choice, and I've learnt not to take it personally if they prefer I not be involved.'

On the fun and exciting side, Broni has been able to assist with the care of close friends she sees regularly, and goes on to watch those babies as they grow. 'Being their midwife is a pretty special relationship to have with these babies and their mothers.'

Broni has also found that sometimes it's stressful in her little hospital not having the backup of a tertiary hospital. Like the day the set of tiny twins were born.

Handover was a bit of a blur that day; Broni can't remember if it was because the ward was unusually busy or she'd just tried to avoid being the one to care for a labour so far out of her comfort zone. She can remember hearing that the fixed-wing aircraft was arriving at 4 p.m. to take the very premature babies' mum to Newcastle. But four o'clock passed and Broni could still hear the woman labouring in the birthing unit. She can remember the doctor saying the mother was ready to push and knew that the rural hospital was soon going to have to care for extremely premature twins. Broni quickly did the maths. Three junior midwives, one senior midwife, one nursing supervisor, one doctor and one registrar for three patients: two prem twins and a mother at risk of bleeding because of her blood pressure problems. Broni didn't think it was enough people (she trained in a tertiary hospital where dozens of people are available to help), and remembers feeling too inexperienced and nervous to be in a situation like that. So instead she 'kind of went into autopilot', pulling a second resuscitation trolley into the room, checking it over just like she would do for a normal birth. Assembling everything they were going to need. Changing all the equipment to the smaller sizes. Getting an oven bag and plastic wrap ready to keep the tiny babies warm and moist (yes, plastic wrap or oven bags with a hole in them for the head are still the best way to keep a tiny prem warm. Staff can tear a hole in the plastic if they need to access an arm, while keeping the warmth in). 'I hunted out the smallest beanies and booties we had.'

When the first twin was born, a little boy, he came over to Broni's resuscitation trolley and the senior midwife began to inflate his lungs with oxygen through the mask. Broni put on the oxygen saturation probe and watched his tiny chest move up and down. 'After about forty minutes we took him out to the nursery and I took over the CPAP.' Broni held the CPAP (continuous positive airway pressure) mask on the baby's face and kept his lungs minutely inflated between breaths. 'In the six or so hours that the twins were in our care I felt protective of that little boy. People kept asking me if I wanted a break, but I didn't want to leave him. He had such a strong grasp reflex with his tiny hand wrapped around my pinkie finger. I felt so relieved when NETS (Neonatal Emergency Transport Service) arrived and were able to ventilate both twins and take them to Newcastle.' The paediatrician from the nearest larger hospital was full of praise for the staff.

In the next few weeks whenever she rang for updates it seemed that the little boy was doing much better than the little girl born after him. Then she came to work one Friday to find out that he hadn't made it. 'I am not a naive person, and we all knew that their chances were slim, but it was still heartbreaking. The little girl was still fighting, though, still hanging in there, and that was nice to hear.'

Five months on, that little girl is about to head home on oxygen until her lungs grow and on caffeine to keep her heart rate up. It will be a long and tough road for baby, mum and dad, but she is still growing and fighting every day.

In her first month as a registered midwife in a birthing unit Broni experienced a series of events that put her at a loss, even led to her questioning whether it was her presence that made things go wrong, like some sort of bad luck charm. There was a snapped cord, which is incredibly rare; a very active neonatal resuscitation with only herself as the resuscitator as the other midwife was dealing with a bleeding mum, also a rare situation when the mums are low risk; and an emergency caesarean section after a long labour that she never expected to go that way and which made her wonder if she had done everything she could to help that mum. This is when other midwives rallied around; her colleagues reassured her and told their own stories, reassured her that she'd chosen a job that has tough times, but the rewards were worth it, and she began to feel better. 'And, the amazing thing about this job is the next day you could have the most perfect birth of your career so far, which turns it all around, and you leave work with the biggest smile on your face.'

CHAPTER 6

Midwife with wings

Jillian Thurlow

Jill Thurlow knows the best position in the aircraft to be seated in for maximum access to a patient; she knows the physics of running IV fluids in flight; she knows that as a flight nurse your blood increases its haemoglobin count when you are working at altitude for any length of time. She knows all this without forgetting the human component of where the best seat is for a mother to comfort her child. Jill, previously an emergency nurse, has found special joy in midwifery on her journey to become a flight nurse for the Royal Flying Doctor Service.

The jump from being a highly valued and skilled member of the emergency room team after becoming a registered nurse to learning the mysteries of midwifery had some challenges. As a midwifery student in a large tertiary centre, Jill remembers she enjoyed her rotations throughout postnatal, antenatal high-risk and antenatal clinics, but once she found her feet in the delivery suite, she realised caring for women in labour was her favourite aspect.

Jill found midwifery challenging but incredibly rewarding, particularly with eventful and emotional births; births where everyone in the room including the midwives were in tears as the new mother and father discovered for themselves the gender of their new bub; births where the women only just made it down the hallway into the delivery room before their baby was born; births spent supporting a terrified teenager screaming her way through each contraction, and the stressed soon-to-be grandmother. Jill remembers the first time she really appreciated she had midwifery skills as well as emergency skills – it started with a normal day and a low-risk woman due for assessment.

After saying hello, Jill learnt that Nell, a woman a few days away from her due date, was in possible early labour and had been brought around to the delivery suite for assessment. Jill explained that while she was a registered nurse, she was a student midwife – she'd take direct care of Nell until she was close to birthing, but would continually refer to the senior midwife who'd be there at the birth to oversee all care.

Nell laughed and said she was pretty sure that wouldn't be happening today, as her three previous babies had all been 'brought on' for being well over their due date, and her husband, who worked away in the mines, couldn't be there for a week.

Jill sought out the senior midwife, involved several rooms away in an imminent birth, and passed over the admission news, then went back to start the paperwork and assessment of her new patient. On her return, Nell told Jill she was really keen to use the bathroom. Just a niggle of unease made Jill hesitate, but she couldn't notice any obvious signs Nell was actively labouring – no complaints of regular contractions, she'd not broken her waters, and she seemed to be lying on the bed comfortably.

'For some reason I just had a gut feeling and explained to Nell that it was better to be safe than sorry, and I wanted to have a neonatal resuscitaire in the room just in case. Nell laughed and said that was fine, that she often worked on Murphy's Law herself, and in this case would be thrilled if she birthed quickly for once.'

Pushing the emergency trolley for babies into the room, Jill checked the equipment while she heard about Nell's three children whom she'd just dropped off to school, and all Nell's post-date induction labours, with no complications or post-partum haemorrhages. Nell hadn't brought in her antenatal history, and no notes had been brought in from the day unit yet, so it was all useful information. Nell had been having an irregular backache but was partially distracted from her body's messages while getting her children ready for school; as soon as they'd been dropped off, however, she couldn't ignore it.

Now they had emergencies covered, Jill was happy to assist Nell into the bathroom. During this time Jill's educator Toni came into the room. Toni was the kind of midwife Jill aspired to be. She gave Toni the quick rundown on Nell's history, and information such as wanting to breastfeed, wanting to have a drug-free labour and an active third stage (in other words, happy to have the injection that helps the placenta to be expelled more quickly), wanting immediate skin-to-skin contact at birth and slightly delayed cord-clamping.

Just as Jill finished handover Nell appeared at the door of the bathroom, leant on the frame and breathed out heavily. She focused on the bed, forced herself to walk across the room to lean over it, and ground out, '*I need to push.*'

They pressed the buzzer twice for another midwife to be present for the birth (it is standard to have two registered midwives at a birth) but things were progressing so quickly there was only time for a quick scoot onto the bed for Nell so they could feel the baby's position, a glance under sheets at a baby's head just on view, and preparation of the birthing set-up. They pushed the buzzer again, Nell pushed her baby, and within a moment the baby was born. Jill lifted the impatient baby onto the mother's chest and glanced at the clock for time of birth, and they all drew a breath.

Nell's baby, stunned for a moment after such a rapid birth, responded quickly to a firm rub with the towel and the sound of his mother's heartbeat. Baby lay on Nell's chest and they waited for the cord to stop pulsating prior to clamping it. Toni had given the Syntocinon – a drug to assist with the separation of the placenta and decrease the incidence of bleeding after birth – and again they double-buzzed for assistance.

It's worth mentioning here that babies love to surprise you and often when you expect help, and even if half an hour ago the place was quiet, help doesn't always come because everyone has their hands full of suddenly arriving babies.

Nell's placenta slipped out complete, which was great, but her uterus didn't contract afterwards as it should have. Nell began to bleed heavily, a wide pool of bright blood forming as she gushed and gushed and gushed, despite Jill's attempts to slow it by massaging the fundus. Toni triple-buzzed this time, the standard hospital call for emergency that ensures priority response. Another midwife arrived, switched off the buzzer, and was asked to draw up 40 units of Syntocinon (which also helps contract the uterus) into a bag of intravenous fluids ready to be continually infused.

Jill rubbed Nell's abdomen more firmly, feeling the bogginess of a uterus that should have been hard like a lemon under the skin but instead felt like a soft grapefruit – loose and floppy. 'You're having a little bleed, so while we rub you should continue to enjoy that gorgeous baby of yours,' she murmured, thinking this was like ED all over again, in that basic ABCs needed to be watched as well as reassuring the patient as emergencies unfold.

Toni checked the placenta hadn't broken and left pieces behind, one of the reasons a woman bleeds after birth, as the blood continued to pour and Jill quickly inserted a urinary catheter, as sometimes a full bladder can stop the uterus contracting too. It was then Jill realised Nell had no cannula in and they were short of hands to put one in, so Jill grabbed a large-bore cannula and inserted it into Nell's hand, securing it quickly before returning to rub the fundus. That done, the midwife could connect the Syntocinon infusion, and they triple-buzzed again for more assistance.

Jill nudged the baby closer to Nell's nipple in the hope it might begin to suckle and assist to slow the bleeding – a baby at the breast makes the mother's body release the hormone oxytocin, which contracts the uterus. This is why mothers breastfeeding soon after labour often get 'afterpains' (Syntocinon is the synthetic version of oxytocin).

As Jill rubbed the fundus, which was still not firm, she noticed the IV line pulling at the cannula and requested some more tape – something she would do ten times a day in the ED with an agitated patient but isn't so common in maternity to have to worry so urgently about an unsecured cannula, but the movement was instinctive and rapid. She continued to massage the fundus with her other hand as she retaped the cannula securely, taped the IV line onto the woman's arm as an extra anchor, asked how she was going and commented again how beautiful her baby was.

It was then she noticed Toni looking at her with approval. A little embarrassed at the attention, Jill murmured the potential causes of a postpartum haemorrhage and its solutions: Tone, Trauma, Tissue, Thrombin, rub the fundus, commence Syntocinon, empty the bladder, look for trauma or pieces of placental tissue preventing the fundus from contracting . . . then noticed the bleeding had pretty much stopped. Phew.

Now the fundus was firm and central, the catheter was draining, Syntocinon was running into the vein at the correct rate to help the uterus stay contracted. Nell, oblivious to events, was getting acquainted with her child, and suddenly called out, 'Oh my gosh, it's a boy!'

All of a sudden a team of doctors and midwives responded to the second bell and arrived to assist. Seeing the woman gazing at her child, and Toni and Jill standing nearby, they looked baffled and asked if they had the right room. Toni laughed and said, 'Yes, but Jill's got it all under control now.' Jill's pretty sure she went bright red, but was secretly thrilled to have proved useful. Combining ED nursing and midwifery worked quite well.

Birth is not always a drama, and many births turn out the way everyone hopes. Jill remembers a couple she was able to follow all the way through their pregnancy early in her midwifery career. To make it even more special, this was their first full-term pregnancy; the mother had miscarried a child at ten weeks, then had to resort to IVF following years and years of trying to become pregnant.

Jill remembers at her first antenatal appointment the mother had nervously asked when she could have an epidural. Everyone had laughed when Jill quipped she had one out the back if she wanted one now, before making sure she sent her new mum-to-be home armed with information on epidurals, to consider the benefits and negatives so they could discuss them next visit.

Information is plentiful and Jill finds it reassuring how well-informed women are for their decision-making around labour and birth, and that the midwifery students, fresh from university, are pushing the boundaries of the latest best practice.

The next time Jill saw this couple, the mother had changed her mind about having an epidural after some reading and research and now wanted to talk about waterbirth instead. Over the weeks they discussed all of her options, Jill building a rapport with the husband, always the joker, and the woman, who always wanted to know what was best for her child.

Fortunately Jill was on shift when this lady turned up at the hospital, labouring beautifully with four contractions every ten minutes. 'That rapport we had became invaluable as I supported her throughout her labour. I knew her requests and her knowledge base regarding the options.'

Because of this connection, Jill could reassure the husband and assist him, her hands over his, to birth his beautiful baby boy onto his wife's chest. To have him involved like this had been one of their dreams, and while the two of them shared a tear as they became acquainted with their child, Jill did her best to stop her watery eyes from doing the same. 'It was such a special experience, and so lovely to be able to fulfil their wishes. It may sound like a cliché, but my passion is sharing knowledge that gives the power back to the woman.'

Now, two years later, Jill laughs, and says the most challenging aspect of her career as a flight nurse/midwife is having to hand the women over to the midwives at the hospital. She wants to stay and provide continuity of care. 'That's what happens with midwifery. It sucks you in.'

Being in such an isolated environment up in the air is both

wonderful and challenging for Jill, because while she has time to provide support to the woman and observe her closely throughout the flight, she always has to be prepared for things to change and have a backup plan, as there's no one to come running if she needs help. And a thorough handover from her departure point is essential.

Jill says that as a flight nurse/midwife you have to be a generalist, be adaptable, and have a sound understanding of both the pathophysiology of flight and what usually happens when these new mums arrive at the unfamiliar place they are en route to – information that can empower the mother for her arrival – and, adds Jill, 'Some dedicated TLC never goes astray.' She also feels privileged to fly with the neonatal intensive-care teams around the state and support them in caring for the neonate while in the air.

Funnily, never in her wildest dreams had she envisaged being a midwife. Joining the RFDS was something she decided on later in her nursing career, though she has always been passionate about providing care to those in rural areas. 'Postcode should never be a determinant of what health care is accessible.'

After a few years of being a local hospital delegate for the NSW Nurses and Midwives Association, NSWNMA, and promoting adequate patient–staff ratios, Jill was voted onto the NSWNMA Council to advocate for improved staffing within emergency departments around the state. She soon realised that not only did her passion for providing the best care to her patients lie in advocating for safer nursing ratios, but it also led her to dream of caring for those mothers who don't have all the specialty services five minutes down the road. So she focused her sights on the RFDS, and midwifery training became essential.

Jill feels her midwifery training at a tertiary hospital was well rounded. The hospital had an extremely busy postnatal ward, so she was thankful for all the time-management skills she'd developed over more than four years working in the state's busiest emergency department. That experience helped her on the days the world went crazy and the labour ward staff had to manage an influx of women and babies all at the same time – half an hour between births would have been nice. Her training hospital had a high-risk antenatal ward, a dedicated theatre for caesareans or risky instrumental births, up to fourteen delivery rooms and five birth suites, as well as an assessment unit, high-risk and diabetic antenatal clinics, plus several low-risk antenatal clinics throughout the region feeding into the hospital.

She says it was through this whirlwind of experiences that she developed her passion for midwifery. While grateful for her emergency training, which gave her the ability to stay calm in an emergency, and her general training, where she'd learnt to use an 'across-the-room assessment', she realised she had so much more to learn from midwifery. Like most midwives, she loves expanding her knowledge and skills to support a mother, whether she be a healthy low-risk woman or one with a high-risk pregnancy. Within her role as a flight nurse/midwife Jill further draws from her union experience, advocating for the best interests of women when she briefly assesses a woman in the ambulance prior to loading onto the aircraft.

Jill only spends the occasional shift in birthing now, as a casual midwife, but believes those days help in her role as a flight nurse/midwife because she never knows when to expect a maternity patient.

A typical day starts from an initial page, when she calls in to find out the destinations ahead. Once at work she packs the plane with the gear, makes phone calls to the various hospitals for handovers on the patients they will fly to retrieve, informs the pilot of the patients' weights and discuss any issues they may encounter; for example, which patients may require stretchering up a ramp onto the aircraft, which can be an issue in bad weather. Then they calculate an estimated time of arrival, and get going.

The flight team can be re-tasked at any minute as the day brings more urgent cases. Jill remembers one day they had just handed a patient over to the ambulance service and taken off for the next destination when the satellite phone rang. It was the coordination centre asking them to go to a P1 (priority 1) for a labouring woman in a small rural town with no midwifery or obstetrics services.

While the registered nurse at the facility was doing a fantastic job supporting the woman, she urgently needed backup as she wasn't a midwife. On the way there, Jill received a quick handover from the RN over the phone and asked a few questions regarding her patient's obstetric history to ensure she could be best prepared. Jill expected to meet the woman at the hospital so she could assess her progress via a vaginal examination, which the nurse wasn't trained for, and ensure birth was not imminent. With her equipment ready – Doppler, birthing kit, cord clamp, Syntocinon and emergency medications in case of bleeding after the birth – Jill was as prepared as she could be.

When they landed on the grass runway, Jill and the pilot noticed a woman leaning over the fence concentrating on her breathing, accompanied by an array of at least ten support people. Apparently the medical officer at the hospital had decided it would be for the best if his patient waited at the airport ready to board the plane. This was a very small rural town with no terminal or hangar, only a tiny shed about the size of a backyard aviary to keep a stretcher in. There was definitely nowhere to privately examine the labouring woman.

As a flight nurse/midwife, you always have to be adaptable. So Jill introduced herself to the woman, explained to her husband she needed a minute with her in private and escorted her onto the plane, where she found her to be well into her labour with only a few centimetres to go. The baby's heartbeat was normal and the mother was breathing her way through the contractions, swaying herself from side to side and bearing down a little, involuntarily. The woman panted, then said firmly, 'I am not going to have this baby until I get to town.' Jill knew it would be close, but she also knew it was only a twenty-minute flight to the regional centre; with this baby being the mum's first, Jill had confidence they had time to get her there.

Jill only had to look at the pilot for him to commence his final check of the plane, and she ushered the husband quickly on board to safety-brief them both. The flight seemed longer than twenty minutes, with the time broken into heavy breathing, and hoping this baby would wait. When they landed in the regional town following a turbulent flight that nobody had time to notice, the ambulance was waiting for them. A few minutes later, as Jill was escorting them into the hospital, the mum began to involuntarily groan on the ambulance stretcher as the birth became imminent.

They arrived just in time. During handover to the hospital midwife, one of Jill's friends, Jill received an urgent page for another transfer. She had no choice but to wish the birthing woman all the best and feel terrible about having to go. Of course, throughout the rest of the day her mind was distracted, wondering how they'd got on. As soon as she had a chance, Jill followed up with a quick call to the hospital. She learnt the baby had been born only minutes after she had left, but that everything had gone smoothly, and Jill asked the midwife to congratulate them for her. A few days later she received the most beautiful email with several photos, thanking her for her support. Despite having their hands full with their gorgeous new addition, the grateful parents had taken the time to thank the crew from the RFDS.

Jill understands now that prior to becoming a midwife she had lots to learn about pregnancy and childbirth. Now she looks forward to sharing that information with women, and what she really loves is seeing that she's helped a woman to become confident in her own knowledge and decisions, and if she has been with a woman during a transfer to a major centre, that she feels more prepared for the coming hours.

During her midwifery training Jill was exposed to so many experiences, some fantastic, others challenging and a few very sad; however, every one of those events assists her today to provide the best support she can to the women in her role as a flight nurse/midwife. Jill absolutely loves working with the RFDS, as each and every day they fulfil the organisation's motto of providing the finest care to the furthest corners of Australia.

CHAPTER 7

Emergency retrievals

Priscilla Turner

'Quite honestly, for me, midwifery was a requirement for the job that I do now. I didn't aspire to be a midwife. This view changed when I spent time with women in the Torres Strait. Everything up here is different, and midwifery, often during urgent transfer, is no exception.'

Priscilla Turner works out of far north Queensland as a flight nurse for the RFDS. There are many communities that don't have midwives, and the flight nurse may be the first person on the scene with the skills to be able to help remote mothers have the best outcome possible for their baby.

This was first brought home to Priscilla when they picked up a young mum from Thursday Island who was actively labouring with a gestation of 23 weeks. The chances of such a premature baby surviving, or surviving without major damage to lungs or brain, are small, and very much smaller if born outside a hospital with a large neonatal intensive-care unit (NICU). Due to the mum's early labour and her distance from a major hospital, there had been numerous discussions about the low chance of survival this baby really had, if born before arrival.

To make it even more tragic for these parents, the mother had suffered a miscarriage around 20 weeks' gestation the previous year. She desperately wanted this baby, and the doctors had even performed a cerclage – put a stitch into her cervix to try to keep the bottom of her uterus from opening prematurely again – but her labour had started and things were rapidly progressing for her.

Unfortunately there are only a certain number of neonatal intensive care beds available in each state. These beds fill quickly with little patients who may stay for many months, so they are prioritised for the babies who have the best chance of surviving.

Townsville NICU had been involved with the calls during the day, hoping a neonatal bed would become available, until finally the night consultant made the call everyone had been waiting for. If Retrieval Services could get this mum down to Townsville before birth, the consultant would do everything she could to give this baby the best outcome. Everything went into hyper drive from there.

The RFDS team flew with two flight nurses and a doctor, which is an unusual configuration; usually it is one flight nurse, and less rarely one nurse and a doctor. Priscilla was finishing her final check-off as a new flight nurse and was accompanied by her nurse manager at the time. She was still working in the special care nursery at Townsville Hospital as a midwife, so they decided on the way up that should this mother birth during the flight, the nurse manager would care for her, Priscilla would manage the baby, and the doctor would support both as needed.

To Priscilla's surprise, when they arrived in Thursday Island, she recognised the woman from the time she had worked in TI while doing the rural and Indigenous section of her midwifery training the year before. So at least there was a tiny decrease in stress for the mother, seeing a face she knew and trusted.

'I'm a firm believer that a baby feels what Mum is feeling and that a mother has the power to control her labour to a degree,' Priscilla says. She was able to sit with the young mum and talk about scenarios and possibilities and what the mother could do to help her baby. The mother needed to know that while they would do their utmost to get her to Townsville where she and the baby could get the care they'd need, if things progressed to the point of no return, they would have to divert into Cairns.

The mum began to cry and said that the doctors had told her that if she had the baby on the way, the baby would not be able to survive until they landed because of his early gestation and requirement for respiratory support by an experienced NICU doctor, which they didn't have.

She and her husband had agreed that she would kangaroo cuddle the baby – that is, cradle baby's bare skin against mum's skin so the tiny newborn feels the warmth, smells mum's scent, and hears mother's heartbeat until the baby's own heartbeat finally slowed and stopped. That heartbreaking fact acknowledged, the mother added, 'Should my baby make it to Townsville, I want to try everything to save my baby.'

Priscilla told her she understood, that they desperately wanted to get her to Townsville intact, so she encouraged the mother to talk to her baby and to believe with all her strength that she would make it to Townsville. This very determined mother calmed herself as much as possible in order to slow the contractions to give her baby the best chance at life.

They took off, everyone holding their breath. It was the quietest flight Priscilla had ever been on. The three staff barely shifted in their seats, let alone spoke, extremely conscious of not distracting the mother concentrating on slowing her labour. The entire crew marvelled at how this mother's contractions had decreased in strength and become less frequent, although they never completely stopped. Occasionally, the pilot would check on how things were going and a whispered voice from the cabin would repeat the instruction to continue heading for Townsville as fast as he could. When they reached the point where the aircraft either turned for Cairns or continued to Townsville the decision was made to keep going, as the mum was still winning over her labour. For Priscilla, 'The last leg was the longest thirty-five minutes of my life.'

As they touched down in Townsville, as if released from a spring, the mum's contractions began to increase. They hurriedly loaded her into the ambulance, jammed everyone in and tore off for the hospital. Mum's contractions built stronger and became more frequent the nearer they got to the hospital, and she barely managed to arrive with her waters intact. After a rush through the corridors they were met by the NICU team in the birth suite, and within minutes of being transferred to the bed the mother birthed a beautiful baby boy. Suddenly her baby's chances of survival had been greatly increased. 'So a very tense flight, but very much worth it in the end,' Priscilla says with satisfaction.

To Priscilla's delight, this little boy, Scout, proved to be amazing. She was still working in the special care nursery and was able to watch over him on her shifts there in the next weeks and months. He did well for the first few days and then his condition deteriorated until his little body was close to a multi-system shutdown. He just stopped coping . . . his obs all started to fall and they were having to support everything, his breathing, blood pressure, etc. His father was a lineman up in the Torres Strait and when urgently contacted he came down to visit his son as quickly as he could. Priscilla remembers that when the dad arrived, the NICU staff gave him what could have been his last cuddle with his baby. However, Scout suddenly stabilised and began to grow again.

It became very obvious that he had a special bond with his dad. Every time he had a bad turn, Dad would cuddle him, talk to him through the cot walls or over the phone if he wasn't back home, and Scout would start fighting again. Scout was in the hospital for about six months before he was discharged to go home with his parents. Despite his low gestational age,

Scout had no deficits to speak of; his hearing, sight and brain function all showed positive signs of being normal. Priscilla remembers him as a beautiful baby who turned out to be quite a fighter thanks to his mother's determination she would make it to Townsville to give her baby the best chance.

Because of her job, Priscilla sees women in all stages of pregnancy. Mostly it's a high-risk scenario such as threatened premature labour or preterm rupture of membranes (which is when a woman's waters break well before the baby's due date). When these women live in remote areas they need to move to a tertiary facility hundreds of kilometres away from home for care in case they go into labour and their baby is born early. Then there are the women who have had an unexpectedly premature baby in a remote area. In those cases, the NICU team will often bring the mother back with them if she is stable enough to fly. Otherwise, another aircraft will go out to retrieve her but it may not be the same day. It depends on the circumstances with the baby and the mother. Occasionally, if the baby is too unstable, the team may not want the mother to fly.

The most typical day involves a call to retrieve a woman in preterm labour. They fly to wherever the woman is, evaluate her to ensure she is safe to travel the required distance, and then off they go. In flight, Priscilla chats with the mother about anything and everything. Often it's a one-on-one conversation, though she remembers many wonderful conversations with mothers and their partners. There are almost always questions they either didn't have time for, didn't understand the answers to, or were simply afraid to ask, and they open up in-flight. 'Maybe because it's just us on this little plane, maybe because they think it's their last chance before they hit the big hospital. I hope it's also because they feel comfortable talking to me. I do my best to answer their questions and to offer some encouragement during the short time I have with them.'

Besides the discussion side of things, Priscilla's primary role is to monitor mother and baby to ensure they arrive safely at whichever hospital they are destined for. Most of the time it's an uneventful flight. Occasionally it's a bit more tense, and she's had another very close call since the premature birth of Scout; thankfully this mum made it into the ambulance before she birthed, so they had more hands and everything went 'spectacularly well'.

Priscilla feels very fortunate to have done her training with some very experienced midwives who were strong in their practice and tried to pass that on to their students. Midwives who emphasised the concept of the power of the mind, and who have been backed up since by the times when Priscilla's seen women 'control' their labour, for lack of a better term; on the other hand, she's noticed how women can obstruct their labour if their emotions and thoughts are jumbled and not in the right state of acceptance. 'Until you see it happen first hand, it's hard to understand. If I have a lady who's close to losing the plot, I use this knowledge from my early midwifery mentors to talk through what their fears are, suggest what resources they have, and help them gain control again. The mind can do amazing things with the body. It's like Scout's mum – she focused so hard on being calm and having a calm belly that when she reached Townsville and relaxed, things completely changed from how they had been for nearly two and a half hours.'

Priscilla is another midwife, like Jill and Glenda, who says one of the most challenging areas of midwifery for her is the access to services. She sees women who have to be moved hours and hundreds of kilometres from their homes and families to birth or await birth many weeks later. Most mothers don't complain, accepting this situation because of where they live. They seem to be so adaptable to it all, but Priscilla says, 'It doesn't mean that we shouldn't be working towards changing things so this doesn't have to be their norm.'

Her stories epitomise the joys of emergency retrieval midwifery, and underscore the importance of establishing rapport while keeping the mother and her baby safe in that short window of transferring them to a higher-care facility.

Midwifery has captured Priscilla's heart and she remembers a special first-time mum at forty-two years old. This mum had laboured at home for as long as she dared, while hoping the labour would stop, because her husband was working away and she wanted him home before she went into labour. By the time she'd arrived in the hospital there was no doubt she would have her baby that day. She had her best friend there as her backup support person and Priscilla remembers the calm, quiet mood of the room, the lights down and the music on. Mum was waiting for her husband to arrive. He had started to head for home as soon as he heard. He had called several times, but it became very apparent he wasn't going to make it before the birth, and Priscilla remembers how the tension increased.

The mum was upset and kept saying she didn't want to have this baby without him. With the change in mood, the pain increased, and Priscilla noticed that the mum had begun to sweat. The mum's friend recognised this too and they both tried to calm her.

The woman's friend was amazing. She reminded the mother they knew this might happen and that's why they made a backup plan. She told her she knew she was a poor replacement for her husband, but she would be there for her every step of the way. Priscilla suggested they call her husband and put him on speakerphone for the birth so he could be there with them.

So with mum standing, and the bed raised as high as it would go with the phone set in the middle of the mattress, the two friends linked wrists across the bed. The mother went on to have the most beautiful birth standing up, holding on to her best friend, with her husband's voice offering support the whole time.

Priscilla's philosophy for midwifery is simply midwives helping women. 'It has to be about *that* woman, the one you are with right then, and what they envision for their pregnancy. We have an obligation to educate women and to give them the tools to make informed decisions, but from there on it's their decision, so we need to be unbiased and non-judgemental in care. We must advocate for them in vulnerable moments so they aren't taken advantage of, and we need to support them in their stronger times as well. Midwives should be the ones they feel comfortable talking to about any questions, concerns, fears or worries, and we should be able to help them through those times. We have to set aside our own feelings, opinions and prejudices and be there for *that* woman when it is her time and help her to achieve the best outcome. I think that's what the role of a midwife is.'

CHAPTER 8

Remote island midwife

Annie Delaine

Annie Delaine is one of those calm and quietly confident women who manage people with diplomatic efficiency and then glide away to the next crisis not just outwardly unruffled but inwardly centred. When the invitation came for me to visit Annie and hear about her work, amid the white beaches and blue-green water on Thursday Island, it was too good an opportunity to miss. I spent a few days with Annie and her husband, Chris, in the Torres Strait, and came away inspired. What I love about Annie's tale is the understated brilliance of what these remote area nurses are doing on the very edges of Australia. The island of Saibai, where Annie has been working the last two years, provides magnificent emergency care for not just those born to the Torres Straits but also those who come across in small boats from neighbouring Papua New

Guinea. Without people like Annie, and her colleague Teresa, and the health workers on all these tiny islands, lives would be lost. Some still are unable to be saved, but not without a tenacious fight from people like those in the team on Saibai.

'I remember clearly deciding when I was ten years old that I was going to become a nurse and wear a veil,' Annie says. 'It seemed no time at all before Mum was picking me up from high school to go for an interview at our local hospital. The matron asked me, "Why do you want to be a nurse?"' Not being experienced at interviews, Annie hadn't even thought about what she might be asked – she could hardly say, 'I wanted to wear a veil.' But she got the job.

That was in 1972. While training, Annie was exposed to labouring women and the birthing of their babies, and was fascinated and intrigued. She almost had to beg to be allowed into the delivery room and then had to stand against the wall, hands behind her back, to witness the miracle of birth. Soon after graduating as an enrolled nurse, a position sometimes limited by its less senior roles, she grasped an opportunity at the Loxton District Hospital in South Australia's Riverland for a student registered nurse position. The matron only hired 'double certificate sisters' – registered nurses who were also registered midwives – so it was a natural progression for Annie to further train as a midwife after completing her general nurse's training.

Nineteen seventy-seven was a big year for Annie. She

graduated as a registered nurse, married a Loxton boy, Chris, and headed to Queensland for a twelve-month honeymoon while she did her midwifery at the Royal Women's Hospital in Brisbane. In the seventies that hospital had a large catchment area and delivered around 300 babies a month, with the capacity for complicated pregnancies and deliveries, and proved an interesting place to train.

After Annie completed her midwifery training, she and Chris returned to Loxton to live, and started a family of their own.

Annie muses that she became a better midwife after having children herself, mostly because the emotions experienced during pregnancy and the tumult at birth helped her to comprehend the complexities of the experience for other women. Then again, she's met fabulous midwives who've never had children, and others who have a brood yet miss the point in their work. So who knows?

Annie was lucky in labour, having her first little girl in four hours. Her second little girl was born while she was on duty. Annie was working her last scheduled shift on Easter Sunday afternoon when she began to have contractions. This wasn't supposed to happen – she still had three and a half weeks to go. She was the only midwife on in the hospital and, it being Easter, she couldn't find another midwife to come in and help; such are the joys of working in small communities and having limited backup staff. However, the matron had rostered on another registered nurse, who turned out to be brilliantly adaptable. She was able to set up for the birth and assist the night duty midwife who came in early for her shift, so in the end Annie didn't have to catch her own baby.

Annie worked in the rural hopitals in Riverland as a midwife and also in the operating theater for many years. She then went on to be director of nursing at that small South Australian hospital complex for ten years, for a while running a small Bowen therapy business as well. When their children were grown she and her husband decided they needed a change, so they rented their house out, and set out for Cairns with two cars and a camper van. Annie became nurse manager at Cairns Red Cross for ten months, then moved on to Thursday Island to be the director of nursing there for over a year.

It sounds easy moving from one workplace to the next – just hitch up your van and travel – but there's nothing easy about fitting into management roles, creating cohesion in teams and smoothing change in the workforce while always keeping the best practice and patient care front and centre in your mind. But the real challenges came when Annie heard the call of more remote nursing. She thinks it was probably watching that helicopter take off and land from the red H on Thursday Island every day, wishing she was aboard. So she and Chris moved out to Darnley Island in the Torres Strait for two years to work with the Erub people, with Annie as their remote area nurse.

After two years on Darnley, of being on call nearly every night as the only nurse 90 per cent of the time, of missing many beautiful dinners cooked by Chris because of a medical crisis like chest pain, child convulsions, the threat of an outbreak of communicable disease or even a terrible toothache, they needed a break, so they moved on again. This time they worked their way around Western Australia, with Chris making a living via his plumbing and maintenance skills, and Annie filling nursing posts for holiday relief.

They zigzagged up and down the huge expanse of Western Australia, through Shark Bay and out on the Abrolhos Islands. During a stint in the Kimberleys, working at Wyndham Hospital, Annie suffered a nasty fall while climbing over rocks that almost cost her ability to walk. She was stretchered out of Emma Gorge on a spinal board, the precursor of months of recovery from the fall and an operation and spinal fusion.

Returning to the eastern side of Australia Annie again found herself drawn to the Torres Strait. There was something magical about the blue-green waters and smiling people that drew her back. Perhaps she ate the fruit of the wongai tree, which, legend has it, means you will always come back to Torres Strait.

Annie and Chris settled on Saibai Island, a 6 by about 22-kilometre island that is mainly mangrove and muddy wetlands with a small village on one end. During the wet season only about 10 per cent of the island is water-free, while through the dry season around 50 per cent is not damp, but still has plenty of waterholes and mush. In fact, Saibai is sinking into the ocean, and has been for years. The cemetery is slowly falling into the sea and the graves are threatening to float away, so the authorities are busily shoring up the edges with retaining walls. However, it is a thriving community of over 370 souls, with a local council, a school, a shop, a pub, and the primary health centre where Annie works. Police, Immigration, Customs and Quarantine also have offices there.

Saibai is a part of Queensland, though Annie's friends and family often say to her, 'When are you both coming back to Australia?' It may be Australia, but there is only 4 kilometres of water between Saibai and the Papua New Guinean mainland and on a low, low tide, a sand and shell dry bar appears about 2 kilometres out (a place where Chris has caught many a fish dinner in his boat to bring home) – this is the border between the two countries.

Those born on Saibai are a proud people, with a long history and deep ties to their island. Their culture is family oriented, and their complex family dynamics can sometimes be difficult to understand from a Western perspective. Family ties are strong and extended, and children are well loved.

Torres Strait has fifteen islands with primary health centres, and another five clinics on the northern peninsula of mainland Australia, for the Aboriginal and Torres Strait Islander communities there.

On Saibai, the PHC is a single-storey building only a few years old, but already stretching at the seams with the workload of chronic and emergency health needs of the Saibai islanders and the usually dramatic but transient needs of the Papua New Guinean tribespeople who often arrive unannounced. Radio contact with PNG works poorly most of the time; calls come via a CB radio patched into a Telstra connection, so the quality is bad. Many PNG villages have no communication facilities at all.

The clinic sits only 150 metres from the waterfront, but is not easy to access from the sea because the boat ramp is a few kilomentres around the corner on the other side of the island. On the health centre's side it's all mud and slippery rocks to the ocean when the tide is low, but those from PNG manage the tricky transfer of injured loved ones from whatever small boat carried them from their mainland to the little clinic.

The clinic on Saibai is managed by the Torres Strait Islands health worker allocated to that role. It has two permanent full-time nurses and two advanced trained Torres Strait health workers, but it is rare that these clinicians work an eight-hour day, especially if someone requires air transfer to Thursday Island. Often it's twelve or eighteen hours as they wait for retrieval teams to take the seriously ill in to a centre offering a higher level of care.

The work is constant, challenging and often a little too exciting. Tropical disease treatment and emergency patients are unable to be fully managed on Saibai, but people arrive day and night for emergency care. Tuberculosis, malaria, taipan snakebites and accidental and not-so-accidental trauma are not uncommon, but some of the most life-threatening cases are the women who are brought over in small boats from PNG in labour or having just birthed in the bush, or with sick babies.

Apart from the nursing staff, there is a doctor who visits every three weeks for three days, and outreach teams fly in to assist with the management of antenatal women and chronic disease. Saibai PHC relies on telecommunications; video links with specialists can be accessed, and telephone advice is available as needed. But until help arrives, the hands-on nurses and health workers are it.

Annie has hundreds of stories of emergencies managed on Saibai. I can only hope that one day she'll write a book on the many lives that have been saved by the clinic on this tiny island, but here I've concentrated on the ingenuity and gritty determination of her midwifery.

Annie estimates there are on average six pregnant women living on the island at any one time. An outreach midwife flies in from Thursday Island once a month, and the pregnant women fly for scans and birth to Thursday Island or Cairns. In between they are managed by the clinic, but the bulk of Annie's maternity workload comes from PNG in little boats.

As the midwife on the island, Annie manages a great number of unplanned antenatal, labour and delivery cases, plus the challenge of premature and sick neonates. She rarely sees her Saibai mothers in labour, as they fly out a few weeks before their due date to await their births.

Annie has one or two premature or sick neonates arrive on Saibai every month from PNG, having been born in the bush, their umbilical cords tied with vine runners and cut with any sharp object off the ground. Depending where they come from they may be anywhere from twelve hours to some days old. They're often too sick or small to suckle at the breast, are cold and wet from the boat ride across to Saibai, and are not always breathing well.

Thankfully, Annie says, the mothers usually arrive in pretty good physical shape, but often they're understandably terrified their baby is dying. Sometimes they are.

Annie tells the story of Hermis, a premature baby she met after a disjointed radio call from the health worker at a village across the water in PNG.

'Baby coming . . . boat . . . *crackle crackle* . . . dropped . . . bad head. *Crackle crackle* . . .'

Annie smiles. 'It was almost a relief when the baby arrived and we found it wasn't injured from an accidental fall, baby had never been dropped, but rather because it was eight weeks premature and the long labour had shaped the head to look misshapen.'

The baby boy was in need of fluids, sugar and most definitely warmth. When managing babies the rule is pink, warm and sweet, and young Hermis was blue, cold and needing some glucose. 'We set about warming Hermis and giving IV access, taking blood samples and liaising with doctors on Thursday Island, who gave us fluid orders to rehydrate and give much-needed sugar to this little boy.' I loved the way Annie said this, as if it's easy to place an IV line into a cold 32-week baby's tiny veins. Believe me, it isn't easy.

'His temperature slowly increased until his heart rate and breathing improved, and we knew we were winning. We waited for the helicopter, doctor and paramedic to come and collect Hermis and his mum to go to Thursday Island and then down to Townsville.'

I'm pretty sure it was a little more complicated than that.

Plus it would have taken a while, and Annie would have philosophically waited for the sound of the helicopter as she kept the baby stable, watched over the mum, and hoped nobody else in need of help came to the clinic door in the meantime. Often they did.

After a few weeks of stabilising and growing and fattening up, Hermis and his mum were flown back to Saibai before they headed home. They called into the clinic to visit Annie, who was hardly recognised little Hermis as the wee scrap of a baby she'd seen the month before. He was now a chubby, healthy and happy baby boy . . . and very much alive, with no 'bad head'. So Annie waved them back into their tiny boat, back across the water, back to the bush, where Hermis, Annie had no doubt, would grow to become a fine hunter. For Annie it was an amazing yet humbling gift to have been briefly in his life. For me it is an incredible story of human caring leading to survival.

Annie talks of another morning, a warm windy day with leaves blowing across the road, from trees so different to those in southern Australia, where Annie is from.

This particular morning, an obviously labouring woman and her husband arrived from PNG. As with most PNG ladies, Annie remembers the woman had a high pain threshold, and didn't complain. This was her sixth pregnancy, and she had five children. The mother had known something was wrong because her strong contractions were very close together but the baby wasn't coming. As her husband said, 'This one's not right.'

Though the mother spoke very little English, she was able

to indicate that she believed her baby was due the next month but she hadn't felt it move for four to six weeks. Annie has often found it difficult to confirm dates and times in these situations, because dates and months are not important in the PNG culture.

When Annie examined her she could hear no fetal heartbeat, nor feel any movements, and the growth of this woman's uterus was about four weeks less than it should have been. Plus the baby's position palpated as breech, a position more common earlier in pregnancy, so that in itself was a hint as to when the baby had stopped growing.

Sadly everything pointed to the fact that the baby had died at least a month before. When Annie felt inside the mother she found the baby was definitely coming bottom first – and soon.

Immediately, Annie knew this delivery could become complicated – the risk of bleeding is high with a baby that has died in the mother's uterus, not to mention the breech delivery – so she quickly called the doctor on Thursday Island to ask him to stand by with the video conference unit. They set up for delivery, and summoned the two staff members available just in time for the poor little baby girl who had died some weeks earlier to make her arrival.

Annie remembers the mother remained very stoic and believes she had known of her baby's passing for some time. She declined to hold her baby, but did look at her tiny face and say goodbye. The father, who had quietly disappeared for the birth according to tradition, equally mysteriously reappeared and was visibly shaken by his loss. He gently cuddled his little girl for as long as possible. The doctor didn't make the video conference in time to help, but luckily this mum didn't bleed too much after the birth.

Annie created a coffin from a foam esky, in which clinic drugs were delivered at that time, and laid the child carefully in it. Her little body felt very fragile. 'That was when I cried.'

As a midwife and clinician, needing to be a leader in an emergency, to be thinking ahead and directing staff who are not trained in midwifery or obstetrics on what to do next, your own emotions need to take a back seat.

Annie sighs. 'I know the fate of this little girl was sealed some weeks earlier, but there was still a sense of failure and emptiness in my heart as I handed the mother and father their baby in a foam coffin to go back in the boat across the water to another country before it was too dark to travel.'

As I listen to this story and blink back my own tears, I think that for this family, there was a blessing in the care they received – the respect for the parents, the safe birthing of the mother, the gentle handling of their precious daughter. It makes me proud that there are midwives out there providing this service. That despite the cross-border issues and need for these people to be on their way home to their own country as soon as possible, our government does support that emergency care from people like Annie and the amazing young doctors, nurses and ancillary staff I met in my time on Thursday Island.

But that particular breezy day didn't end there. Annie said she had the feeling it was going to be one of *those* nights on Saibai. As a remote area nurse on the island, of course you need to be able to manage anything that comes through the door, not just mothers-to-be and their babies. Because this day had been extra busy Annie had headed home late, while her colleague Teresa was still on duty with a patient.

Annie shakes her head as she remembers another call from PNG. 'Patient coming . . . *crackle crackle* . . . Head hurt. Much blood . . . *crackle* . . . Please help.'

So Annie put down her fork, looked longingly at her dinner, and went with the security man/ambulance driver to the waterfront to collect the patient. While waiting for the boat to reach the shore, she heard the familiar sound of a four-wheel bike coming down the road; it was one of the Saibai islanders with his very pregnant PNG partner balancing precariously on the wheel hub – and of course they were heading for the clinic. 'That's when I knew I wouldn't get back to my dinner tonight.'

The first patient arrived by boat and they took her back to the clinic. She'd been beaten by her husband, who had attacked her face with a broken ceramic cup, and was in a bad way. Annie handed her over to Teresa, who needed the only treatment room to care for her. Annie focused on the pregnant Papue New Guinean woman and took her to the consulting room – a much smaller space, but it would have to do. The mother was already established in strong labour, baby coming headfirst, all other parameters good, so following discussion with the doctor on Thursday Island, it was decided she'd have to deliver at the clinic.

This isn't always the case. If in early labour, and providing all the assessments are good, the woman is usually asked to return to PNG to birth. If the labour is well established or at night, and it's therefore unsafe for a mother to travel back in a boat across the water, the family stay at least until morning. If she is more than 4–5 centimetres dilated, the option of helicopter medivac isn't feasible because of the risk of delivery mid-flight. This woman was even further along in labour, so she went ahead and delivered in the consulting room of the Saibai clinic.

Approximately once a month a woman from PNG gives birth on Saibai. Annie stands by as she births, makes sure she and the baby are fine, feeds them and bundles them off home again. The women sometimes turn up because they've had something happen in the past, or have a concern, so often there is a complication for Annie to deal with or refer on to Thursday Island if there's time.

At about two in the morning Annie's mobile phone rang beside her bed. It was the health worker whose phone was connected to the emergency buzzer at the PHC.

'There's a lady at the health centre having a baby.'

'Okay. On my way.'

Quietly, trying not to wake Chris, Annie got out of bed without turning on the light and felt for her clothes. From habit, she always has them out on the chair ready to go for emergencies. Trying to hurry, she nearly fell over when she heard the yelling and desperate banging on the door.

Bang bang bang. A man's voice: 'Baby coming. Baby coming.'

That's it, Annie thought, *Chris is awake anyway*, so she

switched on the light and asked her husband to run downstairs to let the poor man know she was coming. Arriving at the door seconds later, Annie found a very anxious father waiting, and heard the cry of a baby coming from the porch of the clinic about 50 metres away. Annie's first thought was *Good Apgar score*. 'Baby sounds healthy,' she said reassuringly to the new dad. 'Congratulations. Let's go and see what you have.'

At the porch of the clinic, they found the mother lying on the decking with a rag covering her and her baby. Two female relatives hovered nearby. Annie flipped back the covers, reassured herself mother and baby were doing well, and whipped inside the clinic to fetch some warmer wraps and equipment.

By now the health worker had arrived from her house, and Annie was able to clamp and cut the cord and get mother and baby inside to give the woman a Syntocinon injection and wait for signs of separation of the placenta – all normal stuff.

The poor mother and Annie finally had a chance to introduce themselves to one other in the light. The woman was apologetic. 'Tried hard, but had to lie down as baby ready.' She went on to tell Annie, 'This is baby number nine.'

Surprised, Annie felt the need to ask why she'd come across to Saibai to have her baby when she hadn't for previous births. That's when she learnt this lady had lost a lot of blood in the bush last time, and was frightened. Alarm bells began to jangle insistently.

Annie didn't need to be told twice that there was a big chance of another bleed coming up. So in went two large-bore cannulas, and an infusion to help contract a relaxing uterus was prepared in case. The emergency postpartum haemorrhage pack was set out. A quick test of the mother's haemoglobin levels showed that she was already critically anaemic, with barely half the amount of red cells considered normal, and so already behind the eight ball. She really couldn't afford to lose much more, or she wouldn't have enough oxygen-carrying capacity to stay conscious.

Annie had no choice but to get on with delivering the placenta, which hadn't arrived spontaneously. Of course, after that the bleeding began.

Postpartum haemorrhage is still the major cause of maternal death in third-world countries, and Annie was no stranger to following the lifesaving protocols that aren't available in the bush in PNG. But she was still on an island with only a non-midwifery nurse, a health worker and a security guy, and medical reinforcements a flight away on Thursday Island.

Annie got to work. Rub her fundus, up with the infusion, increase the fluids, more needles and tablets to encourage contraction of her floppy uterus – the most common cause of bleeding after birth, and even more common in a woman with eight previous pregnancies. Put baby to the breast to suckle and help the uterus contract, and assess the four Ts of postpartum bleeding. Tone – floppy uterus not constricting the blood vessels where the placenta had been adhered; trauma – a tear inside or outside the vagina; tissue – just a tiny piece of placental tissue left behind can cause massive bleeding; thrombin – even a clotting problem needed to be excluded.

The uterus finally began to contrac tinto a hardening ball

and, with some deep breaths for Annie as her adrenalin ran overtime, the bleeding slowed after 1.5 litres was lost. Annie would have preferred less, but it could have been worse, and with iron tablets mum would recover.

Annie has no doubt this woman's chances of survival if she'd delivered in the bush would have been minimal. She had support people with her that night in the form of her sissy and aunty, who often helped deliver babies in the village, and they were avid watchers of all Annie did. Both said they hadn't known that putting the baby to the breast and rubbing the fundus of the uterus from outside the belly could stop the bleeding.

With the mother's permission, Annie showed them where and how to rub the fundus that night. All she can do is hope this may help save the next mother they care for, as the number of lives lost in childbirth in the western province of PNG for both mother and baby is very high. There was good reason for this mother to be frightened.

As the sun came up and the bleeding remained settled Annie sutured the mother's perineum, which had suffered some trauma at delivery. Annie offered her a tiny stick in the arm, called Implanon, which gives three years of contraception. Annie's lady readily accepted, and Annie arranged iron tablets to help raise her iron levels. 'When I got her up for a shower she'd never seen one before, and I was grounded yet again – we take so much for granted.' Annie's patient enjoyed the novelty of the shower. 'If a woman can safely navigate the shower test, then she's fairly stable.'

Luckily they had some food in the clinic, as by now the mother, father, sissy and aunty were pretty hungry – so Milo and WeetBix helped fill their bellies. Then it was back to the waterfront, where the water was calm, the father smiling a huge white toothy grin, and baby snuggled into Mum's protective arms as Annie bid them all goodbye.

CHAPTER 9

President, Australian College of Midwives

Caroline Homer

In the small mission hospital in Malawi, Africa, women often laboured alone. Tiny babies with problems had little way of getting the help they needed to survive. For their mothers the aching, terrible grief of loss was overwhelming, as it is the world over. The struggles of these women reminded their young midwife how strong mothers can be – and not just because they walked for hours to get to the hospital, gave birth, rose and washed by perching on a bowl of water on their very uncomfortable trolley bed, and then walked back home with their baby.

When she was twenty-seven years old, and just married, Caroline Homer flew from Australia to Africa to work in a mission hospital in Malawi. Her new husband Greg was paid a small wage as a physician, enough to live on in the village, and Caroline was a volunteer midwife. Caroline remembers it as a defining time. She was in an unfamiliar environment, faced with the fact that babies and women died in childbirth far more frequently than she had realised. This was not something that she'd experienced while training in Australia, and she was terrified. The labour ward was staffed by midwives and students, there were only two doctors in the general mission hospital, and doctors only appeared if you needed to do a caesarean – which meant she learnt a whole lot of new skills very fast.

These days, Caroline Homer is a frequent flyer across Australia and internationally between her many roles, the most recent as the elected president of the Australian College of Midwives. Caroline is a professor of midwifery, Director of the Centre for Midwifery, Child and Family Health, and Associate Dean (International & Development) and Associate Head (WHO Collaborating Centre: Nursing, Midwifery & Health Development) in the Faculty of Health at the University of Technology, Sydney. She also volunteers on the board of Advanced Maternal and Reproductive Education, a not-for-profit body that is focused on education for maternal and reproductive health care providers. Phew. It's all a long way from being a naive young woman working in Africa.

However, the rare days she does manage to work as a clinical midwife alongside birthing women are very rewarding, and she loves that time. For Caroline, it's still all about mothers and babies.

*

Caroline's story starts back in another time of midwifery, and illustrates just how far we've come in lifting the training of midwives and the profession of midwifery in Australia. Caroline began her career as a registered nurse (a qualification she has allowed to lapse to promote the separation of midwifery as a distinct profession from nursing) and graduated as a midwife in 1990 after a twelve-month certificate course at the Royal Hospital for Women in Sydney. While she has the greatest admiration for the midwives who taught her, she's not sure she really 'got' midwifery during her training.

While conceding she'd been a good nurse, Caroline's sense of fulfilment in being a new midwife was not very strong; she suspects she was an efficient obstetric nurse rather than being a midwife – alongside and with women, as the definition goes. Looking at those times from the viewpoint of a professor of midwifery and a mentor for new midwives graduating university in 2016, she realises she didn't understand any of the feminist issues which students are exposed to these days. That is, to be women-centred not institution-centred, addressing issues of gender inequity, power and politics within maternity care, the importance of belonging to a professional college and keeping the needs of the most disadvantaged women and communities at the fore. But that was the nature of the time. Like her fellow midwives, Caroline was a part of the nurses union, but she isn't sure why no one thought to mention that midwives had a professional college – the NSW Midwives' Association – which she only discovered in 1996.

Caroline's training was a lot of fun on a social level, with

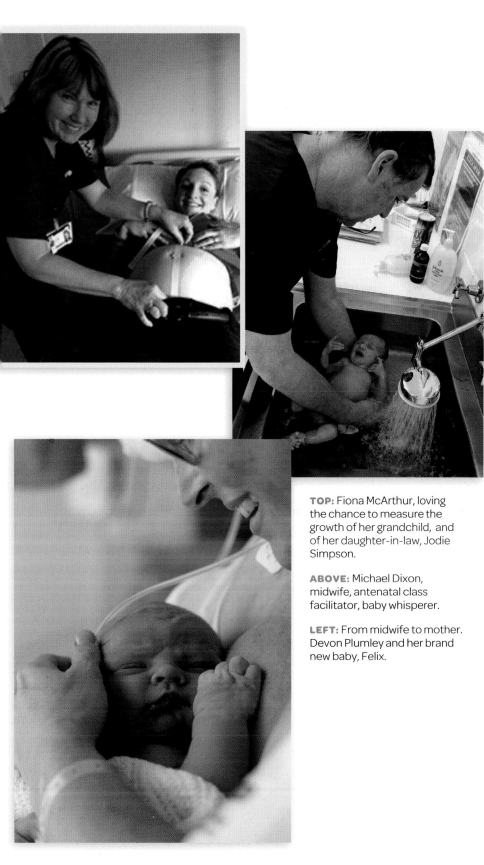

TOP: Fiona McArthur, loving the chance to measure the growth of her grandchild, and of her daughter-in-law, Jodie Simpson.

ABOVE: Michael Dixon, midwife, antenatal class facilitator, baby whisperer.

LEFT: From midwife to mother. Devon Plumley and her brand new baby, Felix.

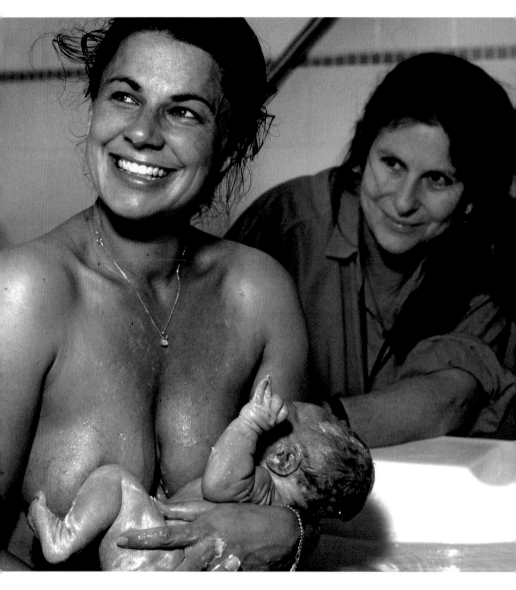

ABOVE: Midwife Shea Caplice is shown in the background of the iconic mother and baby poster from 2000, which helped spread the word about the beauty of women and waterbirth in NSW hospitals. *Image courtesy of David Hancock.*

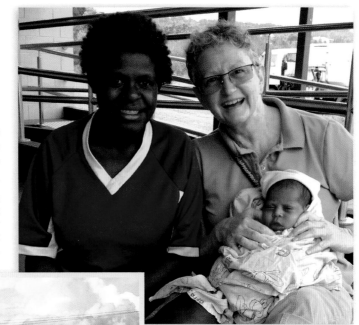

RIGHT: Annie Delaine with a visiting PNG mother and baby.

BELOW: Heather Gulliver's view from the antenatal clinic in Vunapope, looking over the bay towards Mount Tavurvur volcano, PNG.

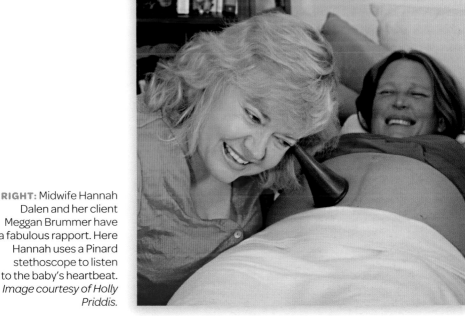

RIGHT: Midwife Hannah Dalen and her client Meggan Brummer have a fabulous rapport. Here Hannah uses a Pinard stethoscope to listen to the baby's heartbeat. *Image courtesy of Holly Priddis.*

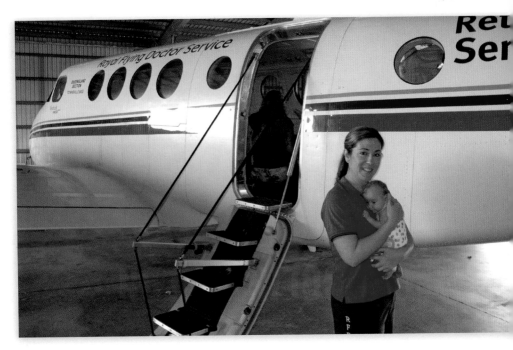

ABOVE: Priscilla Turner with baby Mia beside one of the RFDS Townsville aircraft.

BELOW: Great views are all a part of an RFDS flight nurse's day. This is the view over Horn and Thursday Islands off the Cape, as seen by Priscilla Turner.

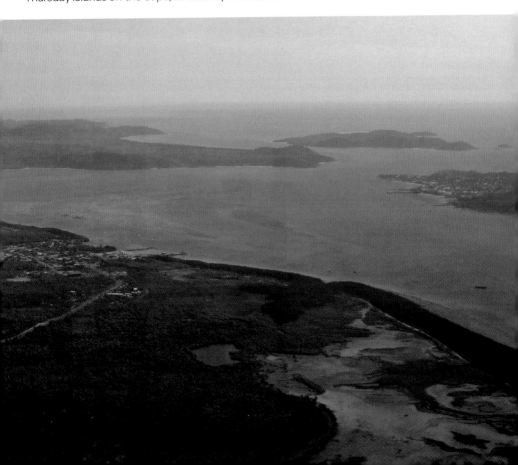

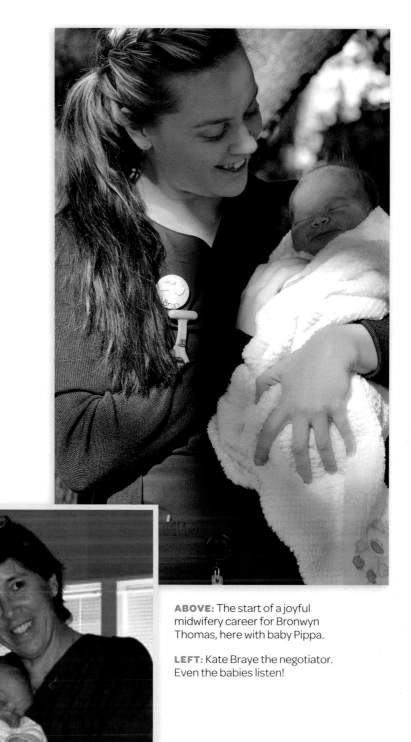

ABOVE: The start of a joyful midwifery career for Bronwyn Thomas, here with baby Pippa.

LEFT: Kate Braye the negotiator. Even the babies listen!

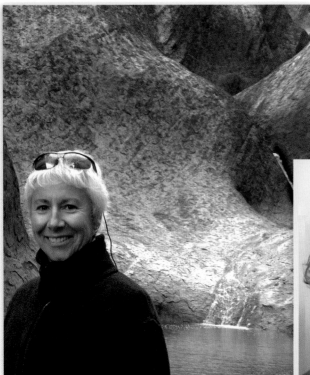

LEFT: When she meets with the Mutitjulu community, Glenda Gleeson is honored to visit the Mutitjulu Waterhole, NT, a sacred women's place and a spiritual area.

BELOW: Kate Dyer, clinical midwife consultant and creator of tiny teddy bears and hats.

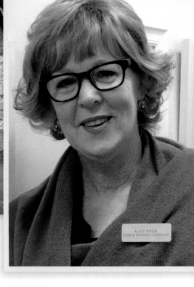

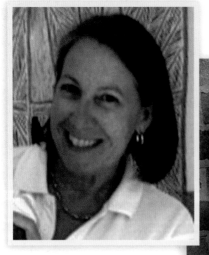

ABOVE: Louise Paul loves midwifery.

RIGHT: Lisa Ferguson, rural midwifery educator, wears the gorgeous Australian College of Midwives 'With Women' pashmina around her neck.

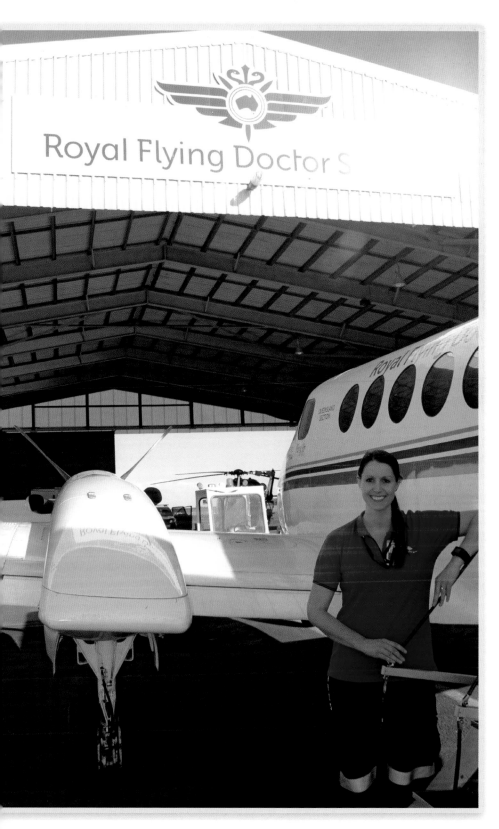

ABOVE: Jillian Thurlow, RFDS midwife in Bundaberg, is ready to fly.

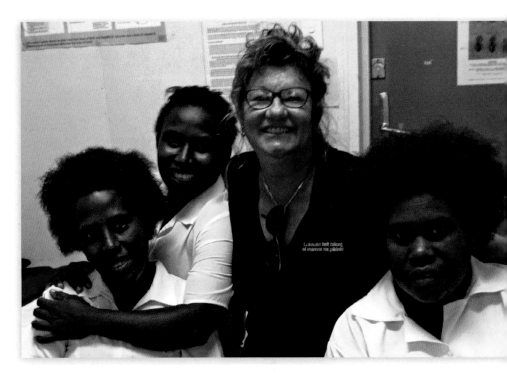

ABOVE: Heather Gulliver with three bachelor of midwifery students from Bougainville, joyfully sharin a moment.

BELOW: Eight of our Aussie Midwives at the Australian College of Midwives Conference, Gold Coast, October 2015. Left to Right: Devon Plumley, Rae Condon, president of the Australian College of Midwives, Caroline Homer, Mandy Hunter, Kate Braye, Shea Caplice, Fiona McArthur, Helen Cooke. *Image courtesy of Photographer At Large.*

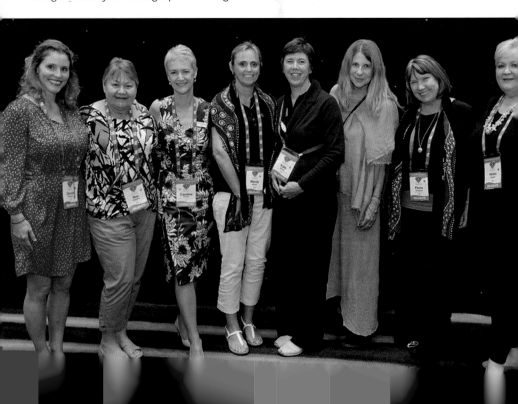

sixty student midwives broken into two groups of thirty for classes. All the classes were held in three-week blocks in the hospital's Nursing Education Centre, where they didn't need to wear uniforms as they didn't see patients, which felt rather special. The uniforms were pale purple stripes with white collars, worn with sensible brown shoes and stockings. Colloquially known as the 'purple morons', it wasn't unusual for the midwives to be mistaken for supermarket checkout operators, who wore similar uniforms.

With less amusement, Caroline remembers her first clinical shift on a Saturday afternoon immediately after completing the three-week theory block. 'Why they thought Saturday seemed a good day to start a brand-new student, I shall never know.' Her first placement was on the high-risk antenatal ward. She'd had no proper orientation to the ward, or even to the hospital. There was herself and a midwife on duty for up to twenty women, all with complex pregnancies. Caroline was shaking in her sensible brown shoes with no idea what to do, having never performed so much as an abdominal palpation or listened to a baby's heart rate. She looks back now and feels very sorry for the women and that midwife, who were exposed to a very green student on a weekend with no other support. 'What were they thinking?'

When people wax romantic about the good old days when nurses and midwives were trained in hospitals and knew how to fluff up pillows and be *real* nurses, Caroline thinks of her training, both as a student nurse and as a midwife. She says there was nothing safe about the way students were thrown in the deep end – and there speaks a woman who is determined that midwives and women are cared for optimally and is moving and shaking to make it happen.

After a number of weeks on the antenatal ward, Caroline was sent to the postnatal ward and allocated twelve women and their babies, even though she had no idea how to change a nappy. Some poor midwife had to teach her these basic skills while chaos reigned around them, as in most busy postnatal wards. Breastfeeding advice and support was a total mystery. 'Who knows what I told those poor women?' It was a baptism of fire, and Caroline can clearly remember worrying if she could ever be a midwife.

Then came the labour ward – a reasonably terrifying experience, but thank goodness for Sister Michie, who is still going strong. She must have taught literally thousands of student midwives in her time. Caroline muses that once she'd calmed down a bit and stopped being terrified of the staff, she realised how much she loved this part of midwifery. She also discovered that things were so much better at night with lots more normal births and a much calmer atmosphere, so she did quite a lot of night shifts.

Remembering the facilities for birthing women makes her grimace. Shared toilets and bathrooms, and small rooms that centred around the large obstetric bed. Each room was a different colour, with matching walls, laminate on the cupboards and benchtops. She quite liked the green and blue and even the maroon room. The worst room was bright yellow and long like a corridor, with the foot of the bed facing the door – so if you entered when a woman was pushing, she was totally exposed. The bright yellow also made a weird optical illusion – as you opened the door, the side-walls appeared to cave in. Caroline smiles. 'I have never seen another bright yellow room in a labour ward, and that is a very good thing.'

At that time and place, it seemed everyone gave birth flat on their back with their legs in the air and staff and doctors loudly urging them to push harder. Enemas were still administered; thankfully, however, shaving women before birth had been phased out.

Caroline is regretful the students never worked in the birth centre, which the Royal was quite famous for. The birth centre was in a cottage separate from the hospital, and Caroline had heard about the amazing midwives who worked there – they even had a bath for birthing women.

Uninspired, Caroline decided not to stay in midwifery, and went off to a job in the children's cancer ward at the Prince of Wales Children's Hospital, perhaps because she felt being a nurse was safer than being a midwife. Although she found her new direction rewarding, it wasn't long before she returned to give midwifery another go in the country for another six months, where she worked on the postnatal ward and in a high-dependency ward in a district hospital. Those few months, helping to make a lot of infant formula every day as most women seemed to be bottle-feeding, were really her only postgraduate experience as a midwife before she went to Africa.

On her first day in Malawi, Caroline remembers the midwives were horrified that she couldn't suture, and could barely take blood or put a drip in. In fact, she'd hardly ever seen a vaginal breech, let alone been the one catching the baby, and of course had never done vacuum extractions – especially with a metal cup and a bicycle pump. The staff were amazing, though, and taught her all this in the first weeks with generosity and good humour.

Greg, who went as a physician, had never done a caesarean, so he had to learn fast – see one; do one; teach one. The first caesarean they did together, Caroline gave the anaesthetic, he handed her the baby and she said, 'It's too small – there must be another one.' Poor man – his first caesarean was twins.

Caroline believes she benefited more from the experience than the Malawi midwives did from her presence. She advises others to acquire skills first and be useful rather than need teaching when you arrive at an outpost.

Soon she was on call for the overnight problems in Malawi. She went in one night because the student on duty thought there was a baby coming with a hand being born first (this is called a hand presentation and means that the baby cannot be born vaginally as the hand, shoulder and head together take up too much space). This complicated delivery would have very little chance of ending with a live baby and the woman could have also been damaged trying to give birth. Caroline immediately called in the theatre team for an emergency caesarean – no mean feat, as someone had to run to the local village to wake the doctor and a scrub nurse and security to open up the theatre. This all took a bit of time at 2 a.m., and the woman continued labouring away. When she was finally transferred to the operating theatre, she gave a big push and two feet came out. Caroline remembers the doctor and nurse saying, 'Oh, great – only a breech,' at which they both turned, left the theatre and went home. Fortunately, it was an easy breech for Caroline and the student – but she always checked before she summoned anyone to open up theatres after that.

There were challenging experiences: maternal and new-born mortality was high; caesareans were done under a Ketamine anaesthetic, which meant the women often had terrible nightmares later on; the HIV virus was just gaining hold, with 10–20 per cent of women being infected and having no prophylactic treatment for their babies; women walked for days to get to hospital; the country was unstable politically, with a president whom her colleagues were frightened to speak out against; and, perhaps most challengingly of all, Caroline had little of the local language. The staff all spoke English, but very few of the patients did.

Women laboured alone while their mothers sat outside and waited. There was a lot of shouting and slapping of birthing mothers by the local midwives – it was shocking and real, and still happens in many countries today, when women make too much noise in labour or the birth attendant thinks they aren't pushing hard enough. Afterwards they washed all the gloves and re-powdered them, and all the needles were sterilised and reused.

'When I reflect back now on their practices I'm horrified, but at the time it was just what happened, so an inexperienced little white girl had no chance of even thinking differently.'

Despite all this, Caroline's time in Malawi was a career-defining experience and one that made her absolutely determined to make things better for all women. Later she also worked for two years as a researcher on an HIV trial, where she learnt clinical procedures like putting IV and PIC lines into people who had one precious vein left – a skill that was very useful in clinical practice.

Back in Australia her midwifery took another turn: she began her PhD and took on the role of midwifery consultant. She also began working in the birth centre at St George Hospital in Sydney, where she paired with another midwife to provide continuity of care throughout pregnancy for one or two women a month. Caroline feels she learnt so much during the six years she did this, finally really understanding being with women. She later worked with two fabulous midwives caring for young, very vulnerable women. These mothers were often teenagers or had drug and alcohol or major social problems such as homelessness or child protection issues. They cared for a number of mothers who had their babies removed into care soon after birth, which was a devastating experience for the women and for the midwives. Being part of the system that has to take a newborn baby from its mother and hand it to the Community Services team for foster care was incredibly hard. The grief and sadness expressed by the mothers at this time, even though they knew it was going to happen, affected all the staff but especially the midwives who had got to know the women through pregnancy.

The most challenging area for Caroline at the moment is

her role as president of the Australian College of Midwives. This is a huge responsibility – one that she wanted to take on, of course, but it's not always clear what is the right strategic path to take for the betterment of midwives and women. The politics of maternity care are tough, and the different groups and their interests, needs, wants and desires are often just different enough to be challenging. 'Sometimes it really feels like we're going backwards, and then other times we can see how far we have come. At a personal level I want to do my best in this role, but I also know that my best might not be what everyone likes or thinks is best.'

Caroline doesn't have typical workdays or weeks as she teaches, leads research, worries about her staff working in Papua New Guinea, attends meetings on all manner of issues, mentors the team she works alongside, supports research students and project staff, and always tries to stop in the middle of the day to have lunch with the team. She also travels frequently – within Australia for the ACM or NHMRC (National Health and Medical Research Council), among others, and internationally to places like PNG and Iran for midwifery development work. The last few years she has been going to PNG up to six times a year depending on the projects. 'When I go there I try to support the midwives, help them problem-solve their challenges, work alongside our PNG colleagues and support them to build their own capacity.'

Her vision for midwifery globally is to work with others to improve the system so that every woman in the world has access to skilled care from a midwife who is educated, regulated and professionally supported. Working on *The Lancet*'s Series on Midwifery and the State of the World's Midwifery report has helped develop this goal, and she is now working with WHO and the International Confederation of Midwives in different countries to help realise it. Caroline believes this will take a long time as so many more midwives need to be educated, but highlighting the goal and the solution is an important step.

At a national level, Caroline's goal is for every woman in Australia to have ready access to midwifery continuity of care – that is, the opportunity to have the same midwife care for them through their pregnancy and during and after birth, so that the woman's wishes are always at the forefront. Alongside this, Caroline is pushing for professional support for midwives. Midwives need options, flexibility and creative ways of working, and to feel that they are professionally nurtured and able to combine a satisfying career with a safe and happy home life.

Caroline's tireless work is helping to shape the evolving world of midwifery in Australia and around the world as she continues to care for birthing women, just like those inspirational midwives she met in Malawi all those years ago.

CHAPTER 10

From Alice to Katherine

Glenda Gleeson

Glenda Gleeson's midwifery practice has been focused mostly on the Northern Territory, from Alice Springs to south of Katherine. It doesn't seem far if you say it quickly – just two girls' names, Alice and Katherine – but try jumping in your dusty car on Monday and coming home Friday, travelling a thousand-kilometre stretch so that you can touch base and offer medical services for Indigenous women in remote and isolated Australia. This was Glenda's way of life for a long time, and she's clocked up the kilometres.

More often now Glenda flies across the country, as a midwifery educator in remote and rural areas. I was lucky enough to connect with her through my interest in CRANAplus, the education arm of the Council of Remote Area Nurses of Australia, for which she was running a midwifery up-skilling course that covered issues in remote midwifery care.

Glenda is involved in teaching midwives, nurses, Aboriginal health workers and medical officers about remote area work. Remote area nursing has unique challenges that crop up away from the resources of more populated areas, and in her course Glenda addresses issues of working, living and travelling remote. With about fifteen courses a year, she undertakes a lot of legwork transporting equipment and manuals, organising course numbers and a teaching team, and most importantly delivering the information to answer the burning questions of those embarking on a remote health career. Privately Glenda is also an activist for maternity services for Indigenous women and pathways for Indigenous midwives, highlighting obstacles to those causes.

Glenda started out as a registered nurse with majority experience in emergency nursing. She graduated as a midwife in 1998 in Alice Springs, so she has Australia's centre in her heart. 'One of my greatest challenges in becoming a midwife was the change from being an emergency nurse, with dramatic and wild Thursday-night brawls, to learning instead how to be truly with women during their birthing time.'

The moral of the story for Glenda is that pregnant women are not sick; if they can gain enough control over their fear and strong contractions they can relax, and in that way achieve control over their labour.

'Having worked for a number of years in oncology and emergency nursing, the joy of working with primarily well women and their families as a midwife meant there'd be no going back to nursing for me. Once I had entered the midwifery world, I knew I'd found my place in the health industry.'

Glenda believes herself fortunate to have trained in a unit in Alice Springs which prided itself on being women-centred, with inspiring midwifery mentors. Glenda's passion was ignited by the needs of Indigenous women, and the 50 per cent of her clients who were Aboriginal women in remote areas became her focus.

Attending to and advocating for young Aboriginal women in labour were light-bulb moments for Glenda and her voice softens as her empathy shines through. 'These young women, a lot only sixteen or eighteen years old, arrive at 38 weeks to "sit down". For me, that term is so evocative of a young woman squatting alone as she waits – alone in a foreign place which could be a hostel, a hotel, a hospital maternity unit if she is unwell, to await the birth or receive treatment for a medical problem in pregnancy. Some have to leave their families even earlier, such as at around 36 weeks, because they are ill with pre-eclampsia or diabetes, or their baby is not growing as well as it should. Others are healthy with a normal pregnancy and are simply awaiting the commencement of labour.

How do these young pregnant women make their way to hospital from their remote communities? Glenda's answer is simple and poignant. 'They get on a bus and are driven away from their families.' Centre Bush Bus is a service developed over the last fifteen years that operates all around the Central Australia region. It's a private company that started as one little bus from Docker, and now travels up to a million kilometres a year. Kudos to the wonderful people who run the bus service, but I can just picture an already homesick young Aboriginal woman sitting on her backpack waiting to be picked up, her pregnant belly under her T-shirt, with her sissies and aunties ready to wave goodbye to her. How sad for the young mum that she has to leave her 'country' and all she knows at such an important time in her life.

Glenda never takes for granted the complete trust these young women place in non-Indigenous midwives to care for them, and the way they allow her to share this incredibly intimate space of their pregnancy and birth. It is something that profoundly touches Glenda. Midwifery is a far cry from the emergency department, where she had weekly experiences similar to being in a war zone, with a large number of women and men presenting with trauma due to violence.

We move on to an example of her work, her day, her week as a remote area midwife. Glenda speaks about a young woman of seventeen she met in a remote community five hours' drive from Alice Springs. This young woman was 36 weeks into her first pregnancy, and presented with vomiting and a headache. Glenda's assessment indicated pre-eclampsia, an unpredictable and escalating pregnancy-induced illness that is dangerous to mothers and babies. Glenda began to arrange evacuation to Alice Springs Hospital, but before she could finalise the details the distressed and frightened young woman requested to have the local nungkari (Indigenous healer) treat her in the clinic before she left. Glenda looked to her patient's family to organise this, and the nungkari came to treat her. Glenda found it fascinating that a male nungkari was acceptable for the young woman, because she knew that pregnancy is very sacred, private and strictly women's business for Central Desert women.

Glenda was relieved to see that after the nungkari's treatment the young woman was much more at ease about the transfer, and it showed her the significance traditional healers still have for young Indigenous people in the twenty-first century.

When Glenda returned to Alice Springs some two days later, she visited the young woman in hospital where her labour was being induced. Her mother was with her, and they were very happy to see Glenda. Although Glenda wasn't there for the birth, just being around and supporting them from behind the scenes had a big impact on these people away from their family. The young woman progressed to birth her beautiful healthy baby and soon the little family headed back to their home.

When the young woman returned to her community post birth, Glenda followed her up so the circle of care continued there. A few months later, tragically, the baby died of Sudden Infant Death Syndrome, the unexplained, little understood tragedy of healthy babies dying, to the devastation of all. Glenda remembers it as a shocking event for everyone concerned. The family organised the ceremony in Alice Springs, and Glenda was invited. 'This was a first time for me to attend an Indigenous family's funeral ceremony, and the first funeral of any child whose life I had participated in. These memories are forever with me and keep me focused on our need to work much harder for the needs of Indigenous Australians, to allow them to be who they want to be and birth where they want to birth, because country is so important to their health and wellbeing.'

Glenda advocates for greater access to medical staff and for more visiting specialists, because despite the high level of chronic illness in Central Australia, communities' options for access to specialist care are few and very far between in remote centres. She believes we need infrastructure and system changes around women having to travel to Alice Springs to birth. A step in the right direction would be a continuity midwifery program for remote Indigenous women, so they could at least build rapport with the midwife who would be at their birth.

Incorporating cultural and family needs into at times inflexible maternal health systems is another challenge for all health care providers and policy makers. One of the ways they can foster change around birth for Indigenous women is by promoting the education of Indigenous women to become midwives and experts in developing appropriate maternity services and programs.

I ask Glenda where she thinks she's grown with her experiences, and she says it was in learning to communicate with Indigenous women in a respectful manner, and in a way that enabled the women to understand as fully as possible the medical processes related to pregnancy and birth.

She attributes her learning to the leaders of the birthing unit during her midwifery training who taught her so much about being with women. Sandy, Kym, Sue, Chris and Jenny were passionate midwives and strong communicators with the obstetric medical staff, ensuring the women in their care had the best chance of avoiding a caesarean section. This advocacy was vital when 50 per cent of the Aboriginal women presenting to the unit had English as a second or third language and a very basic education level. 'I hadn't experienced such care and advocacy for clients in a health system in my former life in nursing.'

Many of the women were affected by problems with alcohol, cigarettes/chewing tobacco, or petrol-sniffing and were desperate for compassionate support. The warmth, respect, and insight of health workers who genuinely strive to provide culturally appropriate care is something we find more and more evidence of as we delve deeper into outreach midwifery in remote Australia.

Glenda speaks of a young Aboriginal woman pregnant with her first baby who arrived on the bus to birth in the unit very far from her family and outback community. Her downcast eyes, her trembling fingers, the way she pressed back into the chair with each contraction showed Glenda how very frightened about labour this young woman was. It took all of Glenda's resources to slowly connect and then support and assist this terrified young woman to be active and work with the contractions to progress through the labour. Over time the young woman developed trust and her baby moved down slowly but surely, so that although the labour took many hours, she finally had a normal birth, and was so very proud of herself and so delighted with her beautiful child. 'If it hadn't been for the senior midwives supporting and protecting us, leaving us alone and reassuring medical staff who may have felt impelled to intervene, it would have been different.' A caesarean section when a first-time mother's progress is a little slower than 'normal' is a dangerous thing for a woman who may in the future have many babies, close together, and a long way from health services. A uterus weakened by scarring from a caesarean has more risk of rupture than a non-scarred one.

I ask Glenda about her philosophy of midwifery and her passion. 'That women, no matter what race, religion, education level, and wherever they live, are able to have safe, culturally appropriate and accessible health care.'

It's not surprising that Glenda has a global view of women and birth. During 2006–2007 she worked in a maternal and child primary health facility in Pakistan with Médecins Sans Frontières, an agency that places volunteer health staff, doctors, nurses and midwives all over the world where needed. Working internationally was something she'd dreamed of doing, and it was a fantastic time to gain insight into the Muslim world.

She was based in the south-west corner of Pakistan, near the Afghan border, under extremely high security. Yes, it was challenging, living and working with an international team, bombs exploding regularly in nearby shopping centres. 'But it was the greatest education I could have jammed into nine months.' It was during winter, and temperatures were minus 13–14 degrees Celsius. 'At night you weren't allowed out, so I had to make assessments of a woman's situation via telephone communication from the local health staff.' This was extremely tricky when the local staff had a very basic knowledge of obstetrics, what was normal and what was not. The MSF outpost conducted a twenty-four-hour birthing facility, an antenatal clinic, a community-visiting postnatal program, and immunisation and nutrition programs.

'I learnt quickly how to gain the required information from the staff and to make a decision about management. This was a real challenge during the night, because to consider referral by road transport was precarious for both the women and the staff. The risk of being attacked on the road during a one-hour journey was extremely high. It was difficult to know fully what was happening for a woman as some staff were more skilled than others, as in all health services.' She was on call twenty-four seven for four months before she had a break, a big change from her experience of midwifery in Australia.

Glenda also spent six months in Papua New Guinea on a pilot project teaching the national nurses about midwifery. Midwifery educators selected from New Zealand and Australia were based in Port Moresby, Madang and Goroka, working side by side with the educators in the midwifery schools. They also worked clinically with the midwifery students and the women and babies in very poor health facility conditions.

The program ensured the midwifery educators were buddied up in pairs at each of the universities in the different cities. Glenda shared a flat with Lois, another Australian midwife in Madang. The aim of the program was to develop a relationship with the Papua New Guinean staff and together improve the education program for midwifery and the treatment of the women who come to use health services. Glenda found working to elevate the service for the PNG women, even in little ways, immensely satisfying but demanding. Then life intruded, and she left PNG after six months because she needed to come home to Alice Springs. But her experience there has only fuelled her desire to improve conditions for Australian Indigenous women.

Glenda's vision spells out her yearning for an environment that nurtures and encourages young Aboriginal women towards midwifery as a vocation. Imagine even one young woman from each community being mentored in a collaborative environment, learning with other Indigenous women to meet and overcome challenges so that they can actively support the next new mother-to-be from their own community on her birth journey.

'The workforce of Indigenous midwives, wise in the challenges and misconceptions that can arise from our well-meaning but often blinkered non-Indigenous perspective, is growing – but very slowly.' Glenda's experiences overseas have shown her that the process of creating change and optimum services for women in these outback communities has some similarity to that in developing countries in Asia and the

Pacific but is different due to the layers of complexity unique to Indigenous cultural context.

Glenda says that remote area midwifery has a very unique and special bond within the wider network of professionals. She believes herself incredibly fortunate to know and be friends with midwives who are absolutely passionate and have given a great part of their life to midwifery. For her it is a true privilege to be a part of the midwifery fraternity, to enable Indigenous women to take the optimal pathway to motherhood and new life, and to foster Indigenous women on their journeys to becoming midwives in their own right.

CHAPTER 11

Coming home again

Hannah Dahlen

It was 1975 in Yemen, in the Middle East. Hannah Dahlen was eleven years of age when Fatima went into labour. Amal, her best friend, woke Hannah and along with the local midwife they brought a beautiful little girl into the world high above the flat rooftops of the city. Fatima took one look at the child and turned her head. 'Take it away,' she said, 'it's another girl.'

Fatima's value as a woman and wife was tied to her ability to produce sons, not daughters. Hannah can still remember holding that perfect newborn baby as dawn broke and the first thin warble from the minarets began to break up the quiet night, and knowing this was her calling. They named the baby Hannah. She understood so clearly then as a young girl that midwifery was a way to change the world, and women's rights was the key.

In November 2012 Hannah Dahlen was named in the *Sydney Morning Herald*'s list of one hundred people who have changed the city, described as a leading science and knowledge thinker due to her research and public profile. I've heard Hannah speak eloquently and with fierce intellect of her commitment to the advancement of professional standards for midwives and for equality of care for all women, but her midwifery career began long before she trained as a midwife.

Hannah was born and raised in Yemen, and grew up surrounded by swirling robes and competing scents of perfume and unwashed bodies. Her mother was an English midwife and her father an Australian teacher of English, who, even though he was without medical qualifications, when needed could turn his hand to healing, and with good results.

Occasionally henna-decorated fingers would dart over the edge of Hannah's playpen to pinch her fair cheek and tug, at times none too gently, at her white-blonde hair. Turning her startled blue eyes on the intruder inevitably resulted in shrieks of astonishment. And so Hannah learnt she was different before she learnt who she was, and when she learnt who she was, she was determined to be different.

Her father and mother's love for each other and the Yemeni people was beyond any example she can think of now, and it was their love and acceptance of those who were sometimes unlovable and unacceptable that taught her to have an open, compassionate heart and, despite the odds, to never give up. It was Hannah's experience of watching the way women were treated and their lack of worth in that society that motivated her to fight for the rights of women alongside their health needs. As she grew older she realised these rights are integral to well-being. Human rights in childbirth became her burning passion.

Many years later, when she was given the honour of delivering a keynote address at the 2005 International Congress of Midwives in Sydney, Hannah told the audience that the first fifteen years of her life in Yemen was spent watching and learning the reality that is a woman's life in a country where women have no rights, no voice and no status. She watched her friends get married as young girls, watched them give birth to stillborn babies after days of labour, and then saw the terrible impact those labours left on their bodies afterwards. She watched girls slave at home and in the fields while their brothers were educated, and watched girls sold into marriage like cattle and boys taught to rule their sisters, mothers and wives. It didn't sit well with Hannah.

She learnt early in life that it is how we grasp opportunity and deal with uncertainty that ultimately alters history and advances society. At five she watched the stars from the flat roof of their house in Yemen with her father and listened on the radio to Apollo 11 return from the first manned mission to the moon, the seemingly impossible achieved.

At twenty-five, the dark, looming presence of the Berlin Wall confounded her. One year later, however, the people brought the wall down. She was in the UK doing her midwifery training when the reunification came. With friends she drove from London to Berlin armed with youth, hopes and one little screwdriver to help them retrieve their bit of the wall.

The wall she now faced was no longer invincible; it had huge sections torn out of it. People sat defiantly on it, their legs swinging over the edge. She still has a postcard from that time, with everyone sitting on the wall and 'Imagine all the people' written across it. 'The will of the people is so strong. We must never underestimate it.' Hannah cherishes that piece of wall and even the blisters she obtained trying to chip it off with her screwdriver. She shows her children this small piece of history and talks with them about the dangers of building walls between people and the need to bring those walls down.

Her childhood and those two momentous events made Hannah determined to reach for the stars and fight injustice. The chances we take today are the opportunities we have tomorrow. As a midwife, a researcher, a teacher and a political activist for women's rights, these life events shaped Hannah profoundly.

At fourteen years of age, Hannah saw what true greatness really means. She admits that not much happened in Yemen for a teenage girl; the odd coup and typhoid epidemic brought excitement, but other than that life was fairly ordinary. She had never met a famous person, so was thrilled to be invited to the orphanage that she helped at to meet Mother Teresa, who was visiting.

The day arrived, and, dressed in her finest, she was ushered in with the dignitaries to meet the amazing woman herself. Mother Teresa had not yet been awarded the Nobel Peace

Prize, but she was well known. The first thing that struck Hannah was how tiny Mother Teresa was. She was like a small, vibrating sparrow with piercing eyes.

'When it was my turn to shake her hand, she fixed me with a gimlet eye and I had nowhere to hide – not behind my fancy clothes, not behind my pretence of sophistication and not behind the blush that flooded my face. She took my hand in hers, weathered and worn with hard work, and gripped it with such amazing strength for a small woman. I felt like she had just seen every secret and vulnerability I possessed.'

Behind Mother Teresa, through the door they were to enter, orphans were being herded, with partial success, by the patient nuns. In front of the sea of children stood a row of chairs for important dignitaries. In the centre of the row was an especially grand chair for the greatest dignitary of all: Mother Teresa.

It was then that Hannah learnt the biggest lesson about greatness, and it's one she has carried with her ever since. From the heaving mass of little, ragged, squirming bodies on the floor a tiny but persistent wail reached Hannah's ears – but not before it had reached Mother Teresa's. Turning from the dignitaries she was supposed to welcome, she moved into the room and went not to her important chair, but to the source of that wail. The heaving mass of children hushed as she entered and she placed a hand on a head here, touched a tiny chin there, until she spotted the sorrowful little girl with the persistent wail. Despite being nearly seventy years of age she crouched on the floor and pulled the crying child into her lap. Startled mid-cry, the little girl grew silent and wide-eyed and Mother Teresa began to sing a song and clap along with it, swaying and crooning in a voice that was not perfect by any means, but utterly beautiful in its intent.

The seething mass, the sobbing child and the herding nuns all stopped and the dignitaries shuffled in the doorway, unsure of what to do – Hannah among them. 'Eventually someone took control and we were moved towards our seats, but the big important chair in the middle sat empty – oh, it was so empty.'

Mother Teresa never left her spot on the floor surrounded by children while the ceremony in her honour took place, and Hannah left that day with a lesson that she's never forgotten: greatness is believing in what you do, and doing what you believe, but knowing that it is not about you.

Midwives have the opportunity so often to be with women in a real and unassuming way that facilitates each woman's potential and brings great joy. At the end of the day, a midwife knows she's fulfilled her role when women are filled with pride in the amazing job they have done. That is the privilege: to have such a special role in women's lives.

So, back to where it all began.

After years of begging to be allowed to see a birth, Hannah had her moment when she was ten. She was put in the corner of the clinic where her parents worked, and watched the midwife orchestrate the whole event with great efficiency. Hannah left the event feeling bewildered, excited and full of questions.

Questions like why, every time the woman rose up off the narrow clinic bed, did the midwife instruct her to lie down again? Later in her life, as a professor of midwifery, she researched this very question.

But back to a girl on the brink of womanhood, in a world on the brink of the major paradigm shift of the seventies, when Hannah was part of a birth that changed her destiny forever.

Hannah's neighbour and soul sister was a Yemeni girl called Amal. 'Two people were never so different. She was destined for a life I'm yet to comprehend, while I was destined for a life of opportunity. I have never again had a friendship that was as deep as ours.' Hannah believes there is something about the friendship of girls as they leave childhood behind and enter womanhood that binds them forever. As the portals of knowing and growing open to allow for the major transitions in our lives, we are left vulnerable and imprintable. This is one reason Hannah thinks pregnancy and birth are such important times of growth but also times of vulnerability to trauma.

As young girls, Amal and Hannah would hide in the tiny grain room of Amal's house, which doubled as her bedroom, and when Amal had finished cooking and cleaning for her family of nine brothers, and Hannah had done her correspondence lessons, they would create worlds of possibilities. Sitting on the sacks of sorghum and the bags of rice, they were queens and conquerors. They had lovers and devotees. But outside of that little room they were once again two girls destined for lives that were an accident of their birth.

Hannah taught Amal to read and write in Arabic and will

never forget her friend writing her own name for the first time. Amal taught Hannah more than Hannah ever taught her, but she does remember teaching Amal that she had a right to the footpath. When women walked on the narrow footpaths in Yemen, they were expected to move into the road if a man approached and let him have the footpath. The road was a dangerous and dirty place to be. Hannah would link her arm through her friend's and hold her fast on the footpath with her. It was so hard for Amal to do. Sometimes at the last moment when a man approached she would pull away and end up on the street, laughing as Hannah ploughed ahead. Sometimes, though, Amal stayed on the footpath, and when she did her smile was radiant. Hannah uses this analogy when she talks about the importance of human rights and safe motherhood. Until women have equal right to the footpath of life, they will not have safe motherhood.

It was Fatima's birth that started this story; she was Amal's sister-in-law, married to Amal's oldest brother. Fatima agreed to let Hannah come and be with her for the birth. At sixteen, Fatima was pregnant with her third child in three years. She had two daughters born a year apart, and there was great hope this baby would be a boy. As a result of three years of pregnancy, Fatima was very anaemic and needed regular iron injections. When Hannah approached Fatima's husband to ask him to drive her, as he possessed the only car in the family, he refused, saying petrol was too expensive and she could walk. And so walk they did. At eleven years old, Hannah carried a child and Amal carried a child, and Fatima walked heavily pregnant with shockingly low haemoglobin to get her iron injection. They did it once or twice before she refused to go back. 'No wonder women die during pregnancy and childbirth if they are seen as less valuable than petrol.'

It is no great surprise then that Hannah ended up in health. On top of her mother's midwifery experiences, her great-grandfather had founded the first Western medical training school in Peking; her grandfather, who had a dream as a medical student that he would find the cure for leprosy, years later did this, being the first to use sulphone therapy (DDS or Dapsone) in 1941, after consulting with chemists in Britain who were using it to treat streptococcal mastitis in cows. So you could say Hannah's career path was pre-destined. Her desire to become a midwife remained strong throughout her teenage years and she went to the United Kingdom to train as a midwife after undertaking nursing training in Australia. Probably one of the main reasons she went to the UK to undertake her midwifery training was that her mother was a midwife in the East End of London in the late 1950s and early 1960s. When the TV series *Call the Midwife* came out her mother had sadly passed away, but her mum's best friend and fellow midwife Fiona was able to share this history with Hannah recently when she was in the UK. They went on a pilgrimage and found the real Nonnatus House they lived and worked in years before. Hannah wrote about this in the article 'Call the Real Midwives'. In fact, it was Jennifer Worth herself, author of the book *Call the Midwife*, who opened the door to Hannah's mother and Fiona when they went there to train as midwives in 1959. Apparently Jennifer looked down her nose over a pair of glasses and said, 'I will let the sister superior know you are here.'

'I was terrified,' Fiona told Hannah. 'I thought, what on earth have I got myself into?' Apparently Hannah's mother was doing a good job faking calmness, a characteristic that came to define her.

Hannah returned to Australia in 1991 and embarked on a twenty-year career in busy public hospitals. While she loved her job, she didn't love the way women were sometimes treated and the way they often became victims of a fragmented and highly medicalised system. Hannah realised the fear had crept into her own mind and she'd begun to think of everything that could go wrong before she thought about what could go right. She found herself, often unwittingly, an instrument of the system rather than in partnership with women. 'Slowly little pieces of my soul felt like they were withering and dying.' She takes her hat off to her many colleagues who managed to carve a path of love and trust through a system that is often an enemy to these fundamental requirements for birth. Thank goodness for these amazing midwives.

'The birth of my own children with wonderful private midwives made me realise strongly we are ripping women off in this country. But my journey into motherhood was not an easy one, and I know there is no greater love than that we have for our children.' Hannah is the mother of four beautiful children – Lydia, Luke, Ethan and Bronte. Her arms, however, hold only two children. Her lap belongs to only two. She gazes in the night at two sleeping faces, yet always imagines the two who may have been. She is a mother four times over and she is so grateful for this blessing, for there are many who never get to feel this love even once.

Her firstborn daughter Lydia turned her reluctantly and then ferociously into a mother. But tragedy struck when her first son, Luke, died at two days old in 2002, and Ethan at eleven days in 2003. They were both perfect and full-term, but had a rare genetic disorder that was only discovered after the birth of Ethan, despite an autopsy following Luke's death. When Ethan was born and did not breathe (just like Luke), investigations commenced and continued until his death eleven days later. In 2005 Hannah's second daughter Bronte was born. She came into their lives full of the reminder of life and filled Hannah's arms and heart once more.

In her article 'A Love that Never Ends', Hannah asks, 'How do you survive a broken heart?' This is a question she has asked herself many times since the deaths of Luke and Ethan, only a year apart. How do you survive a heart broken, not yet healed and broken again so soon? 'We survive because there are others we need to survive for – our beautiful daughters, Lydia and Bronte. We survive because of what may be. We survive because as humans we are eternally hopeful in a future we cannot see. We survive because birth and death are forces that move us from the dermis of our superficial half-lives into the deep life-giving marrow of our existence. We survive because that existence has meaning. We survive because not to is a worse option.'

In the last five years Hannah has moved from a clinical role into an academic role and became Professor of Midwifery at the University of Western Sydney. The questioning nature she developed during her childhood appropriately channelled her into academia. In this role she researches and teaches and manages higher degree research students. This has helped her to work for change to maternity care on a macro rather than a micro level.

Hannah is the national media spokesperson for the Australian College of Midwives, and works hard to launch midwives into the public domain and on the radar of consumers, helping to overcome the invisibility of the profession. The ACM has fought a strong and proud battle in making the recent reforms in maternity come true, and Hannah was so honoured to be a part of that moment in history on 1 November 2010 when midwives gained access to Medicare.

However, amid the excitement and full life she was leading, Hannah missed women and babies and realised she wanted to practise during this historical time in midwifery. Jane, Robyn, Melanie (three wonderful midwives) and Hannah formed a group practice together called Midwives@Sydney and Beyond. Later they were joined by Emma and Janine. Most of the births these midwives attend are homebirths. They all became eligible midwives after undertaking a prescribing course to finally be endorsed by the Nurses and Midwives' Board of Australia. This means the women they care for can get Medicare rebates for a proportion of the care provided, and they can prescribe commonly used medications. Hannah continues to work through the quagmire of collaborative arrangements, Medicare red tape and clinical privileging, but they are getting there. Soon their practice will be able to offer women the option of birth in hospital with a private midwife.

A day in Hannah's life is never the same as the next or the previous day, and that's how she likes it. She finally feels she has come home. She has love and trust once again to fill her working life and bring reality into her research, teaching and political life. She is able to watch the amazing power of women when they know their midwives and believe in themselves. She can see how birth can be, and is simply addicted. The greatest role of a midwife, she knows now, is to keep fear at bay and respect women.

'Going to my first homebirth after many years in 2010 was amazing. As I drove through the dark, empty streets I wound down the window and began to chant my mantra, "trust in birth and respect it also".'

In the early hours of that morning a beautiful little girl was born into water and her parents' arms. Hannah was reminded of the first homebirth she'd attended nearly four decades previously when still a young girl. There was peace, love and power there.

She thought later about how safe it all felt. She realised

with wicked joy that she had violated several hospital protocols and policies, but at no time was the care unsafe. The woman took a while to birth her placenta. In hospital a drip and manual removal may have been her reality, but her uterus was well contracted and they waited. The baby crawled its way up to the breast and Hannah didn't touch it for hours. In hospital, would she have had time to sit and watch and wait? The baby was on the small side and a little cold. In hospital it would have been warmed up under the radiant heater and probably given a blood sugar test, but at home mother and baby were bundled into bed and kept the breastfeeding and skin-to-skin contact happening.

As the garbage trucks rumbled past that morning, the baby's father used the internet to find out the exact time dawn would break and, putting his prayer rug on the floor, he faced west and prayed. There was no call to prayer from the minarets like there was at the first homebirth Hannah had attended, but she knew that while it had taken almost four decades, and was a long and at times convoluted journey, she had finally come home.

As the saying goes, 'Homecoming means coming home to what is in your heart.'

CHAPTER 12

Quest for safety

Mandy Hunter

Mandy Hunter's midwifery career began in her first year of high school with a black-and-white film of a baby being born – and the next thing she knew, she was flat on her back with her legs in the air. Faint number one. Sigh. But from that day midwifery became her dream, and Mandy decreed that fainting wasn't going to stop her.

Some weeks ago, in my small rural hospital, we had a very keen fifteen-year-old work experience student visit our ward, a young woman who is desperate to become a midwife when she leaves school. To her distress, she almost fainted during the newborn baby examination when the doctor checked the baby's hips. After hearing Mandy's story I need to find her and reassure her that if she believes in her dream and doesn't give up, she could be a fantastic midwife just like Mandy.

Mandy is a clinical midwifery consultant at a large tertiary hospital and is my go-to person when I need advice on a new guideline of care for women at my small hospital. Her story resonates with me not just because of her personal heartbreak and the way she rose above it, but because she never gave up on her dream of becoming a midwife.

Mandy's mother was a midwife who trained in Scotland, so Mandy suspected midwifery was her destiny. She loved looking through her mother's textbooks, and of course she wouldn't always faint. Would she?

Mandy planned to study her midwifery in Scotland, too, but fell in love just after completing her general nurse's training and moved to Kalgoorlie instead of Edinburgh – and unfortunately there's no midwifery school in Kalgoorlie. Then Mandy and her husband Paul moved to Tennant Creek in the Northern Territory when they were newly married. There was still no midwifery training possibility, but she did love babies, so it was a joy to fall pregnant.

Mandy's twins story didn't just begin when she found out she was pregnant, because that would ignore all the thoughts and dreams that went before. It included the overwhelming joy of being told she was carrying twins; when she was already thrilled at the idea of being pregnant with one baby, twins were just amazing, and she and Paul felt so lucky. At the time, living in Tennant Creek, a small, remote mining town over 500 kilometres from Alice Springs, they were a long way from either of their families, but all shared their joy.

Her lovely GP provided antenatal care, and she was booked to see the visiting obstetrician at 22 weeks – he visited Tennant Creek every month. Not being a midwife yet, Mandy didn't realise that a twin pregnancy was associated with higher risk, and expected to have her babies in the local hospital. Paul queried the need to move to a larger centre like Melbourne for the end of the pregnancy but the obstetrician assured them both quite emphatically that there was nothing that could go wrong that he couldn't handle, and that he would arrange for Mandy to have her babies in Alice Springs.

Soon after that visit with the obstetrician one of her friends showed her a photo of a woman pregnant at term; the woman was huge with twins, so it didn't alarm Mandy too much that she was growing so quickly. Mandy was working as nurse and time was passing. Nothing was wrong.

Which sadly wasn't true. At 25 weeks' gestation Mandy began to suffer lower back pain. Her GP was concerned enough to ring the obstetrician, who of course remembered the only woman with a twin pregnancy in Tennant Creek at the time. He suggested she take two Panadeine Forte every four hours if needed. The next day Mandy remembers saying to one of the nurses she was working with, 'If I didn't know better I would think that the babies were coming.' She could feel pressure inside, and getting comfortable was proving difficult.

On Saturday morning, Mandy was teary and exhausted. Paul, too, was concerned, and took her up to the maternity ward. Reassurance and sympathy was offered, along with a beanbag kindly donated from the ward, so off she went home with some liniment for her back and a sleeping tablet, and tossed and turned all night.

The next morning Paul came to the hospital with her and insisted she see the doctor. A young doctor from Japan, who knew Mandy well, was concerned and admitted her to the maternity ward for observation. The day went from bad to worse, particularly with the backache; the only position that she found semi-comfortable was propped completely upright with her two feet together. She could hear the male midwife on the phone reassuring her mother that Mandy wasn't too big for her dates, just tired. Everything would be fine. Paul, meanwhile, was worried and discussed Mandy flying to Melbourne as soon as possible; he started to arrange this with her mother for the next day.

Paul went home later that evening, and when another midwife came on for the night shift, she popped her head in before handover and said, 'Don't you do anything on my shift, Mandy.' Mandy, wan and tired, remembers looking up at this midwife and thinking, *What a strange thing to say.* Even then it hadn't entered her mind that anything was wrong.

At about eleven o'clock that night Mandy passed a small mucous plug in the toilet and her alarm bells started to ring. It suddenly dawned on her, through the exhaustion of three days without sleep, that things weren't just uncomfortable – something was terribly wrong. The midwife ushered her back to bed and examined her, and found that Mandy's cervix had started to open. The staff sprang into action, calling the doctor, and Paul, to come.

After many urgent phone calls, at 2 a.m. they wheeled Mandy past the ward desk on her way to the airport and she could hear the nurse on the phone talking to her mother. 'Mandy is being flown to Alice Springs in premature labour.'

Paul, Mandy, the midwife and the young doctor were all crammed into the back of a very small plane, with a single humidicrib. The midwife kept telling her not to push, and Mandy would reply that she wasn't pushing but really needed to go to the toilet – a worrying sign of impending birth for midwives trying to prevent a delivery in a plane. She remembers the pilot kept looking back and asking how she was.

They finally arrived at Alice Springs Hospital early in the morning, where Mandy was taken straight to the delivery room. It was the change of shift, and there were many people in the room when the obstetrician arrived. Mandy remembers him saying, 'Ah, polyhydramnios, I thought so,' and she still wonders if he'd had an inkling at his first visit three weeks prior.

He gravely informed Paul and Mandy that the hospital facilities were limited, and that unless she had her dates wrong and the babies weighed 800 grams or more, they would be too small for them to save. Mandy knew her dates exactly: that day she was 26 weeks pregnant. She begged to be flown to Adelaide where there was a neonatal intensive-care unit, but was told there wasn't enough time.

To Mandy, it seemed like she was detached from the scene and watching someone else's drama unfold. She wasn't watching someone else.

Jack was born at five to nine that morning after one push. The neonatal staff took him straight over to the paediatrician, commenting that he was very small, and Mandy registered straight away that they were not going to be able to save her baby.

The obstetrician ruptured the membranes of Mandy's second baby in a gush of fluid that knocked him backwards off the stool and Mandy looked on, distantly calm when she should have been hysterical, and thought, *I'm going to die.* It just seemed like a fact.

The relief from the constant pain she'd suffered for three days was indescribable, though shatteringly empty, because the physical pain had eased but the emotional trauma was just beginning. She knew both her babies were too small; she could hear the staff talking, and could tell by the atmosphere in the room there was no hope of taking her babies home.

Finally the tiny babies were brought over to Paul and Mandy, and she put their little shiny bodies on her bare skin where they lay, warm against her, until they passed away. Jack was 600 grams and Patrick a tiny 500 grams.

She was taken to a single-bed room and, exhausted and in deep shock, she slept. Paul had to roam a strange town all day by himself with no one to talk to until she woke up. Like the sight of Patrick's bruised arms from his rushed and difficult birth, this is another memory that really upsets Mandy.

When Mandy woke that afternoon, she felt isolated by her grief and will never forget how much she appreciated a mid-wife popping her head in and introducing herself – something she is very aware of now. 'She said she wasn't looking after me, but wanted me to know that she was so sorry for our loss and if there was anything she could do to please press the buzzer.'

Mandy remembers being a student nurse on placement in a maternity ward a few years before this and being told not to go into a room where a woman was recovering after the loss of her baby. That's not what Mandy tells students now. As she sees it, nothing anyone could do would have made her feel any worse than she did, and it helped to know that this midwife cared enough to acknowledge she was there. This is something I pass on to my students too.

Paul stayed in the room overnight with Mandy, so they were finally together in their grief, and Mandy's mother arrived the next morning. It was then the three of them went to see Jack and Patrick, and cradled the tiny bodies. Mandy and her mum bathed them, held them and took in every detail they could. It was such a short and precious time for Mandy and Paul to be parents to Jack and Patrick, and they treasured every heartbreaking second of it. Mandy is incredibly grateful for the time spent with her firstborn boys that day, and the photos taken of them.

Mandy's mother had brought with her matching nightgowns which the boys wore until the day they were buried; these gowns are the first thing each of Mandy's further four children wore after they were born. She often thinks how much her youngest son, Matthew, reminds her of Jack. In fact, all six of their children have the same second toe, longer than their big toe. Her daughter, Julie, has really broad shoulders just like the twins did. It is comforting to be able to visualise them in her memories.

Mandy's recovery wasn't aided by the development of an ileo-femoral deep vein thrombosis, a dangerous complication probably to do with the weight of her hugely pregnant uterus and the time spent on an aircraft flying back to Melbourne where the babies were buried. It took her weeks to recover, with enforced bed rest and medications to keep her blood thin.

The grief process was longer and even more painful. Hurt and angry with the obstetrician, Mandy and her GP went to see him a few weeks after the birth, and even then she felt he missed his part in their loss. 'I didn't want or need him to accept liability, just for him to say he was sorry that I had lost my babies.' This is something Mandy never forgets when she meets grieving parents.

The midwives cared, and she appreciated that, but the reality is that caring is not enough. She tells her students that midwives are professionals with a responsibility to know and recognise complications, and they must be advocates for women; perhaps if she had been warned of the possibilities earlier she could have insisted on transfer to Melbourne before it was too late. This is the backbone of her practice now.

Mandy has a theory on emotional pain: that as humans, we can only ever hurt so much; you can't hurt more than 100 per cent and that is the pain level you experience with the loss of a child, 100 per cent. 'I don't believe it is humanly possible for anyone to ever hurt more than I did then. During that time in my life I hurt all over, every single part of me ached and I felt hollow inside. I remember thinking that I would never be able to smile again. For many weeks I couldn't see an end to my hurt or feeling of loss.'

Mandy's cry echoes that of every mother who has ever lost a child, and I remember her words now whenever I meet a mother or father who has lost a child – they keep me mindful as a midwife of the depth of despair a parent suffers.

But Mandy still wanted to be a midwife. Nearly two years later she and Paul had a baby girl, Julie, then moved to another mining town, Charters Towers. There was still no midwifery training available, so she had time for two more gorgeous babies. Finally they moved to Perth, and Mandy could at last apply for the hospital-based midwifery program at King Edward Memorial.

There Mandy found out she was pregnant, due three months after the course started. She was now desperate to enrol, as this was the only hospital-based training left in Australia, so she covered up her belly and went to the interview. In hospital-based programs you were paid a wage as you learned. University-based midwifery is an unpaid, fee-required option, and financially would have been too difficult for Mandy. Once accepted, she booked a meeting with the director of nursing to admit her pregnancy and declare how badly she wanted to do midwifery. Could she please defer to the next course?

The matron proved to be her champion, and Mandy started midwifery training when Matt, her youngest child, was ten weeks old. The timing wasn't ideal, but finally she was on her path, and she employed a great nanny. Mandy slept with

Matt every night to keep her milk supply going and all was well, though extremely busy.

Now, back to the fainting.

While attending her first birth as a student midwife, Mandy fainted. During the next three months at every birth in her training, she fainted. Not surprisingly, she was in despair. It just wasn't realistic that this profession could be for her. The only thing that kept her going was noticing that she stayed conscious further into the birth each time.

Mandy couldn't do her required theatre nurse component for caesareans – something she caught up on later – as she fainted! The good news is that she did finally get over her lapses into unconsciousness. 'I haven't fainted for years,' Mandy reassures me. I can't help smiling.

But Mandy did develop a fetish for safety in birthing during her time at King Edward. 'I was a very good obstetric nurse, if I do say so myself.' Mandy says. 'I never encouraged a woman to birth off the bed and felt my most in control when she had an epidural, a catheter and Syntocinon in progress. Shameful when I think of it. I wanted so much to have everything covered safety-wise.' No doubt this is her legacy from the loss of her twin sons, Jack and Patrick.

When the family moved to Newcastle, Mandy began to work at a tertiary hospital with a birth centre. In her first year there she was a nervous wreck. They seemed so *casual*. She had a fantastic mentor, who managed the birth centre, but the place terrified her until she settled in. There were mats and birth stools in every delivery room. Barely anyone had their baby on the bed.

However, there were fantastic midwives, and the head of obstetrics at that time was Andrew Bisits, a strong believer in women-centred care and an inspiration from the beginning. It was here Mandy stepped away from the fear cycle she'd been gripped in and completed her evolution into the dynamic leader and teacher she is today.

Now, as a clinical midwifery consultant she has a lot to do with policy; she has just completed the district waterbirth guideline and written a learning package to train midwives in safe waterbirth.

So what does Mandy do now that she is well into her career? A lot of computer work. She attends morning handovers and encourages discussion about management plans for complex cases. She constantly looks for ways to improve services.

At the moment, she's looking for a better way to help babies that need more sugar when first born to supplement their first few breastfeeds. The baby who has had a tiring birth, or of a mum with gestational diabetes, or a baby who is less well grown than expected, is at risk of a sudden fall in glucose after birth and babies need glucose to use for energy, keeping warm, and being alert. Mandy heard of a glucose gel being used in the Sugar Babies Study and studied the research and worked with a neonatologist in John Hunter Hospital to develop a guideline that would give mothers choice in how they want their babies to be treated. Some mums are dreadfully upset if their baby needs to be given formula milk, and Mandy believes there should be choice available.

She goes to meetings for the Quality Use of Medicines program, which she finds very informative, and is Acting Chair of the Hunter New England Human Research Ethics Committee, a lead research ethics committee in NSW that reviews the ethical considerations in all clinical trials.

She's on the executive team for the Women's Health and Maternity Network and is the maternity stream leader for her district. Her main focus in this role is maximising resources by promoting district guidelines and consistency in midwifery care – she wants midwives to practise to their full professional scope as much as possible.

Mandy wants midwives to question practice and be constantly improving how things are done, such as sharing knowledge so that all of the area's birthing services are able to offer water for use in labour as a low-risk comfort measure and as pain relief for birth. For some strange reason much more complex scenarios like induction of labour, twins and epidurals require no extra formal training as the use of water does.

Mandy gets involved in policies such as when to call for more senior advice, known as the escalation plan, and values her network with other clinical midwifery consultants around the state. She is often required to comment on draft state documents, and takes this very seriously, along with sharing guidelines for information. She loves teaching and values her time with the Advanced Life Support in Obstetrics and Becoming a Breech Expert courses.

She believes passionately that the universities have it right, and that training through the Bachelor of Midwifery is the way of the future. She champions student midwives gaining experience in the birth suite and beyond because she's grown into a passionate midwife and is very pro natural birth.

Mandy admits that for a long time she preferred to work in medical rather than midwifery models of care, but realises she was afraid of taking full responsibility for the women in her care; it also took her a long time to be able to trust the process of normal birth and not feel hyper vigilant and anxious about possible complications. She remains committed to raising awareness of the increased risks associated with twins, and the dangers of deep vein thrombosis – but she never, ever faints at a birth anymore.

'It's amazing, really. The more I think about birth the more I realise how much nature has it covered. We need to facilitate physiology, not "manage" women – but we must always remain alert.'

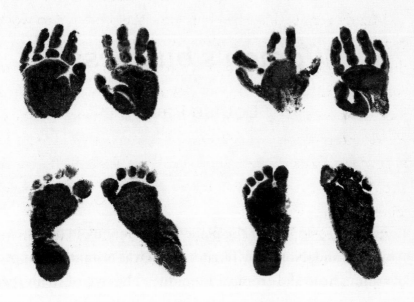

Jack and Patrick – 9 July 1990

CHAPTER 13

Women's business

Louise Paul

Louise Paul stepped off the plane in Nhulunbuy in north-east Arnhem Land, Northern Territory, and was instantly wrapped in stifling heat and tropical humidity. The five of them (her partner, Tony, and their three sons, William, Samuel and James), as well as their Great Dane, Blue, had arrived on the Gove Peninsula aboard the Qantaslink flight – and she only realised how panicked she was when they had to walk down the steep flight of stairs onto the tarmac.

Her three boys were little – William was seven years old and the twins were five. They had no idea what was going on, and certainly didn't know that this was going to be the place where they would grow up. None of them could envisage the dramatic change to their lives. Louise didn't know that her kids' upbringing would be filled with fishing, catching snakes, swimming in croc-infested waters, chasing lizards, camping, riding motorbikes and doing all the dangerous things that kids consider normal when living in Gove.

She was very surprised to see they had to walk at least a hundred metres towards a tin shed that was the airport terminal. They were directed to retrieve their luggage from the vehicle that was used to load and unload the bags. No X-ray devices, no technology.

Looking around, there were two things that struck Louise. One was the incredible ink black of the night sky and the stars that shone like diamonds. 'A clichéd statement, I know, but until you've been here you can't quite understand the beauty of the night sky of Arnhem Land. The blackness is so *black* – it holds such depth, and the stars are so incredibly bright. They truly shine so bright that they light the sky. I have never seen a night sky that is so clear. And I could go on forever about the beauty of the moon.'

The second thing she noticed was the wire fence that separated the tarmac from those waiting to pick up the newly arrived. The fence must have been 10 or 12 feet high, and looked like chicken wire. The people on the other side clung to it, their fingers interwoven in the wire, and everyone called out some sort of welcome to those crossing the tarmac. 'I really felt like I was arriving in the back of beyond.' Later she learnt that the fence was affectionately known as the Wailing Wall. Just a little bit different to the eastern suburbs of Sydney and the Kingsford Smith airport!

Why on earth had she brought her family here?

They arrived at the Top End in December of 2004, during peak wet season, in the hope of rekindling Louise's passion for normal birth and women-centred care. The plan had been to leave behind the disillusionment and frustration of fourteen years of midwifery in tertiary referral hospitals where intervention was normal and 'normal birth' was anything *but* normal.

Louise started her Midwifery Certificate at St Margaret's Hospital, Sydney, in 1990 and had wanted to be 'a good midwife' like her mother. She grew up with birth stories, knew her own birth story – an undiagnosed breech delivered by her aunty, who was an enrolled nurse – and proudly relayed this to anyone who would listen.

Louise knew when each baby of their hometown was about to be born out of business hours, because the same thing happened each time. First there would be a phone call – this was the era of the late sixties through to the early eighties – and their home phone had a very large bell attached to it so the ringing could be heard from the backyard. When it rang it sounded similar to an old-fashioned alarm clock, only a thousand times louder. 'The phone call would always come in the dead of night just when your dreams were at their best.' This would then be followed by her mum's footsteps running down the hallway to answer the phone. Minimal words would be spoken; a short *Right, I'm on my way*. Then there'd be another run back to the bedroom, and within five minutes the back door would be slammed shut, the garage door would be flung open with its loud grating sound, and their old green Holden ute would be given a very loud rev and shoved into reverse down their gravel driveway, its headlights shining for an instant through Louise's bedroom window. Her mum would have hit second gear by the time she was about four houses down and the car would soon be out of earshot. Louise knew it all meant a baby would be arriving soon.

She remembers trying to stay awake so she could hear about the baby and what her mother had done to help the woman and her family. Many of those stories were full of joy and happiness, and some of them were overwhelmingly sad. Louise listened to them in the early hours many times – at a very young age she knew all about not repeating what she was told. By the time Louise reached her late teens, her mum could proudly say, 'See that baby? I delivered her *and* her mother – that's like my grandchild!'

Louise always knew in her heart of hearts that some day she would follow the same path as her mum. 'Mum always had a different look about her when she came home from a birth – I think deep down I wanted that too.'

Then, in her third year of her general training as a nurse, Louise saw her first birth and fell in love with midwifery. She could hardly believe that any woman would be happy to have four student nurses watching her give birth! 'But this most beautiful woman gladly gave her permission for all of us to enter her room, her space, and be part of her birthing experience. I was overwhelmed by her generous attitude. I clearly remember her smiling and saying that it was her fourth baby, and that if it would help us to become midwives, we were more than welcome! I couldn't believe how lucky we were! So the four of us piled into her room, stood at the end of the bed and watched as she breathed and laboured through transition and then calmly entered second stage. She reached down and brought her baby to her chest and greeted it with tears of joy and love, then looked at us and asked *how we all felt*! Can you believe it? I had tears rolling down my face – it was the most amazing and beautiful thing I had ever been part of, and I was so very grateful to this woman. She allowed us to be part of one of the most precious moments in her life. She didn't know us from a bar of soap, yet embraced us as young women trying to find our way in our nursing careers. I knew from then on that one day I would definitely be a midwife. I also now understood what my mother was talking about, and how she felt imbued with light when she talked about birthing. It all seemed to click.'

The most challenging clinical area for Louise is the spectre of sick neonates. 'I fear sick babies; they frighten me, and I worry that I'll fail to pick up on those cues they give us to let us know that all is not well.'

Her first experience of sick newborns was in her second year of general training, when she was sent to children's ICU. She could write a book on the dreadful experiences she had in her eight-week term there! She could also write a thesis on bullying and the everlasting effect it can have on young nurses. Needless to say, for that eight-week period her nights were restless and her dreams were filled with alarms beeping and babies dying. To this day, she still feels traumatised by the treatment of the staff in that unit, and she has never felt so useless and incompetent since. Due to her time at that ICU, when she started midwifery training her biggest fear was that her first ward would be the special care nursery.

The day they were notified of their first placements was nerve-racking for Louise, who couldn't shake her sense of doom. Sure enough, she was devastated to learn of her placement in the special care nursery, and as she'd probably set up to happen, her night-duty introduction to the SCN was horrendous. She was the *only* student midwife on shift, and everyone else may as well have been talking a different language.

Louise remembers the four babies she'd been assigned never seemed to stop crying and screaming, and they certainly didn't stop weeing and pooing. Just as her own tears were brimming, the door of the SCN was flung open and a small-in-stature but larger-than-life woman appeared. Her eyes widened at Louise and the four humidicribs poo-spattered with four screaming babies inside. She walked straight over, asked her name, introduced herself as the night supervisor and began to efficiently feed, clean and sort out Louise's patient load. That was how she met Avis Strahle.

Like a fairy godmother with a magic wand, Avis miraculously made everything better. She broke all the rules that had been laid down to Louise and turned off the phototherapy lights, took the babies out of the cribs and placed them in open cots. Within what seemed to be minutes, she'd scrubbed the humidicribs clean, changed the linen, cleaned the babies and fed the babies. There was still one baby, however, who would not stop screaming. The night supervisor asked Louise to find a cottonwool ball – just one – and hand it to her. Louise couldn't help but wonder what one cottonwool ball was going to do to save the day, but she did as she was asked. Fairy Godmother laid the baby boy on his back, pulled his legs gently to his stomach and ever so lightly (with a feathery touch) tickled him just underneath his testicles. With a wry smile on her face, she said, 'All men like this!' Almost instantly, the baby stopped crying and relaxed, a blissful look on his face. Before Fairy Godmother left the unit, Louise was allowed to have an hour-long break and on return found that she only had two babies in her care. Her fairy godmother became one of her very best friends. But to this day, Louise still has nagging discomfort when confronted with sick babies – not clinically, because she has remedied that with knowledge and experience, but emotionally, because some fears never leave you.

Louise remembers her first delivery very clearly. The senior midwife on duty, Marie Miners who became another treasured mentor, took her by the hand and told her that today was going to be the day she delivered a baby. The labouring woman was a private patient who'd agreed to have Louise care for her, and the obstetrician was a kind older gentleman who was excited to be part of her learning experience. As second stage approached and Louise's nerves started to show, the obstetrician gently covered her hands with his and guided her through the delivery. The baby roared loudly as he entered the world and was placed onto the mother's chest, and everyone cheered. Both the senior midwife and the obstetrician were beaming, and Louise was overwhelmed with emotion. They both hugged her, and once the placenta was delivered and the mum was made comfortable, the senior midwife put her arm around her shoulder and told her to go ring her own mum to tell her about her first birth!

On one of her most tragic days, as a newly graduated midwife working in the delivery suite at her training hospital, she was assigned to care for a woman who had presented the night before. The mother's waters had broken but she hadn't gone into labour, so an induction was started. When Louise started her shift twelve hours later, very little progress had been made. Louise supported the woman in her request for a caesarean section, but the final decision was made without listening to the mother or to Louise.

The night that followed was perhaps the worst night Louise has ever experienced; more importantly, it was the worst night that two people under her care could have ever experienced. That night a baby was lost to the world, and two young people became mourners. This was Louise's first unexpected stillbirth, and it taught her many things.

She learnt that to even more strongly advocate for a woman in her care, the woman must be listened to and her requests and wishes must always be paramount. Her voice must be heard, and if for some reason she cannot speak, then midwives must speak for her. Louise learnt to always document care and events in a very clear and accurate way. If by chance a case goes to court (as this case did), the progress notes will be crucial.

Louise's notes told the accurate story of this dreadful night and cleared her of any wrongdoing, despite the accusations of the obstetrician that the baby died due to poor midwifery care. She learnt how important it is to debrief about adverse events; everyone involved needs to be listened to, everyone needs to be heard. Feelings need to be expressed, and grieving with and for the family – and showing this grief – is an important part of the healing process. And she learnt what it felt like to carry a precious child that cannot stay to his mother, and what a father's primal scream sounds like.

These are memories she carries with her every day.

Even though this story is terribly sad, Louise has many, many happy stories too – happy and inspirational moments that she draws from. 'There's nothing quite like being pulled into a woman's jubilant embrace just after she has given birth while she thanks you for all that you've done. It's difficult to picture a more perfect moment than that of a mother and father looking at their newborn baby in awe and wonder, but it could be when they can still find time in that moment to look at you, their midwife, and tell you they couldn't have done it without you. Then there's seeing a woman for her antenatal consultations and having her tell you that she really hopes you'll be the midwife who cares for her during labour. There is something extra-special about one of your girlfriends coming to you to tell you of her exciting pregnancy news and requesting you to be her midwife. And what completes all this wonder and joy is being able to watch most of these babies grow into beautiful human beings.'

In her early years of midwifery, there was never a time Louise doubted the profession was for her. She loved being with the women and their families, and she loved the delivery suite. Birthing babies was such a special thing that it always brought tears to her eyes.

But what happens when the midwife has her own baby? Is it different from being on the other side? For the birth of Louise's first son, she laboured at home throughout the day. Although she enjoyed being in control at home, there came a point when she needed fresh support and was driven rapidly to the hospital where she worked, fully dilated and demanding an epidural. It was then that Marie Miners walked into the room with the biggest of smiles and told Louise she was going to stay back after her shift to care for her. Louise relaxed and found the space she needed to enter second stage. Her mentor guided Louise and gently instructed Tony, and an hour later the two of them helped their son into the world amid much joy and love and quite a few photos.

Being a midwife did help Louise to anticipate and understand what was happening to her, but she wasn't prepared for the high and elation that birth gives. 'I felt so empowered, so very strong and so complete. My dream of a normal birth without drugs (apart from two sucks on the gas, and a request for an epidural I thankfully didn't get) had come true, and my beautiful friend and mentor had helped Tony deliver our son. What more could you ask for?'

Once she left hospital, though, she felt completely unprepared for what lay ahead. 'Being a mother is the hardest job of all, and there's no real manual that teaches *you* how to be a mother. It's a wonderful journey, and each woman's story is different.'

Louise's second birth two years later was similar in many ways, but also very different. This time around she was carrying twins, and was determined to keep things as natural as her first birth. She didn't want an epidural at all and wanted to have a vaginal delivery. Things didn't quite go to plan, however, as the twins were more rushed than anyone anticipated.

She went into labour and progressed quickly; when she arrived at the delivery suite she told the midwife that the first baby was about to appear. She needed the student midwife to get the camera out of the drug cupboard and stand at the end of the bed taking photos, since her own camera was playing up. By the time she was helped onto the bed, the first head was crowning. The first boy arrived in a hurry, and the second followed after two more contractions. Within ten minutes of arriving in the delivery suite, Louise had had two baby boys, and third stage was completed without incident. It was even more seamless than she expected. When Avis Strahen arrived just after the boys were born, she helped get them on the breast, and when Louise looked around the room at the cast of thousands (everyone comes running when twins are born), she saw her smiling midwife who told Louise she'd just given her the highlight of her career.

Once again, she felt like she'd conquered the world.

Louise started to doubt her career choice about fourteen years into being a midwife. Her passion and love of the craft was leaving her as intervention crept into everything that she and her fellow midwives did. No longer did she feel like she was practising midwifery, but rather that she had become more like the obstetric nurses who did what they were told by the obstetrician. It was induction after induction, epidural after epidural; the majority of births were achieved by some sort of instrumental delivery or caesarean. She wasn't forming valuable relationships with anyone, but was just coming to the hospital, working hard for little reward, and going home feeling unsatisfied. She began to hate working in the delivery suite – the one place she'd always wanted to be. She tried middle management, but that was even worse! She lasted almost three more years, until the idea of washing dishes in a kitchen seemed a viable option for a career change.

Where had her passion gone? What had happened to midwifery care, women-centred care, normal birth and the beauty of being with women? 'I don't think I've ever felt so lost and mentally unwell in all my life.'

Then Louise received a phone call from her brother. He had friends who had just returned from a place called Nhulunbuy, on the Gove Peninsula. He knew that there were jobs going in its small maternity unit and gave her a number to ring. Louise took a deep breath and rang the number, and that's when a magic door opened. 'I did find my passion again among the Indigenous women of north-east Arnhem Land and Groote Eylandt.'

However, her first day on the maternity unit of Gove

District Hospital did nothing to dispel her uncertainty from their arrival on the plane. Feeling anxious and unsure, she tentatively walked onto the ward to find a midwife providing one-on-one care (known as specialling) to a baby in the room they called the nursery. 'Hello,' she greeted Louise. 'I'm Clare, you must be the new midwife. If you go into Room 10 you'll find Sally – she's in charge and will be able to hand over to you. We're waiting for Air Med to transfer this thirty-four-weeker and her mother to Royal Darwin Hospital. We were both called in around five this morning.'

Louise found Room 10, and there was Sally specialling what looked like a very sick woman. There was no high-dependency unit here for this woman, who had had an emergency lower uterine caesarean section for a separating placenta and spiralling blood pressure. With a blood pressure that is climbing dangerously, the blood vessels in the placenta are in danger of bursting under pressure and could cut down on the amount of placenta that is available to keep the baby alive.

'Hi,' Sally said. 'Sorry I can't show you around this morning, we're a bit busy. Will you be right to work on the ward by yourself? Just follow the pathways in the bedside charts and come and check with me if you're not sure. By the way, there are two men in rooms 7 and 8 who need to go to theatre this morning.' Louise's first thought was to run – apart from anything else, she hadn't looked after a male patient for many years – but she bravely headed off to do pre-op checklists and try to reignite her vocation.

On that first day, she learnt that she was a 'yappa', meaning sister or fellow woman in Yolngu Matha; she learnt that the Yolngu style of breastfeeding a baby wasn't documented in any textbook she'd ever read; and that her straight hair was perfect for making rudimentary paintbrushes for the fine crosshatching in Yolngu art. She made up her mind then and there that she was only going to be in this place for twelve months!

Now, a decade later, she's still wiping sweat away in the wet season as a midwife at this end of the Northern Territory, and she can't imagine ever leaving.

Louise loves to tell stories. It's how she teaches others. She loves to talk about her experiences, how things were done when she first entered midwifery, and then incorporate what she's learnt into current thinking and practice. Louise encourages others to tell their stories too. Everyone remembers a good story, and she believes they're a useful path to learning – a different way of teaching, perhaps, but also a way of helping midwives of all age groups and experience levels share for the benefit of all. Louise uses stories in her care of women and their families during all stages of their pregnancies, and loves her work with the passion she thought she'd lost forever before coming to Gove.

The unit she works in now has given her the opportunity to connect with women through their whole pregnancy and beyond. The town she lives in is quite small, so often she sees the women in the shops, or out and about at various social events. 'It's amazing how many consults I've given in the aisles of Woolworths – whether it's about contraception, early pregnancy discomforts or what to expect in labour. Then there are the many chats with brand-new dads who race over to you to ask a question about breastfeeding or growth spurts or why their pregnant wife is so tired. It's fantastic!'

Louise finds that working with the Indigenous women and teenage girls is different on many levels. There is so much to consider. Their lives are nothing like those of Louise and her fellow midwives, and of course there's always the language barrier though she has managed to pick up the most important words. She emphasises that as a midwife you need to be culturally aware, culturally safe and culturally secure.

It's important to understand that the Indigenous women of north-east Arnhem Land will not part with much information – they're shy and frightened and have suffered in many ways. 'This is where my stories help me out! The Indigenous women love stories – it's their way of passing down culture and tradition. They also love picture books. Combine the two, and you can form a relationship. Form a relationship, and you can share information and develop trust. I love it when a woman trusts me and lets me support her and guide her when she needs it.'

So Louise works with women and midwives in the same way. She tells stories of her own experience as a mother, stories about her midwifery experiences, stories about her own life and stories about the lives of others. This helps her to form relationships and work out what needs she should consider and how she can help that person, be it a colleague or a mother and her family.

The days are always filled with laughter and talking and beautiful girls and women who love to talk and tell stories, and when there is a bunch of them together there's a lot of noise! These are days spent sharing information that can help the women, using picture books, DVDs in language, or interpreters. Girls come in from their homelands or outstations for their scans or cardiac reviews or diabetes management. The staff may have two or three women arrive for sit-down, to await the birth of their babies. Reams of paperwork are ploughed through in order to get an idea of their history and any other conditions or chronic diseases. Forms must be filled out, boxes ticked, orientation to ward area given, rights and expectations explained. Risk assessments, skin assessments, referrals to specialists, dental appointments and the like need to be organised. 'It's all about taking the opportunity there and then to treat any condition they may have.' The list is endless: sexually transmitted diseases, scabies and fungal skin conditions, rheumatic heart disease and other cardiac conditions, diabetes, dental caries, malnutrition, chronic airway disease and worms.

Louise could have a busy week with little babies born premature at another hospital such as the Royal Darwin who have been transferred back for fattening up. Mum may need some help to re-establish breastfeeding – this means hours spent expressing, supply-line feeding, tube feeds and demand feeding. Or they could have a very quiet spell with only one or two women waiting to have their babies. The workload can change in a blink of an eye. Like it did a few weeks ago.

Nothing was happening during the day, but by four in the afternoon, Louise and her colleague were looking after two labouring women close to birthing, expecting another labouring mother to arrive from one of the communities via CareFlight, and another sit-down woman had ruptured her membranes. By ten in the evening there was also a baby being specialled on high-flow oxygen, a woman with a suspicious CTG trace awaiting a caesarean section (a cardiotocograph measures contractions and the baby's heart rate, and can help to flag when a baby is becoming distressed and may need intervention), and another woman labouring. Staff were doing overtime and the place was humming!

The scenario was very different at the beginning of the week when one of the women elders from another village wanted to make some bush medicine for her sixteen-year-old granddaughter who had just given birth. She needed an axe to remove bark from a certain tree, and a fire, along with a large bucket of water to soak the bark. Certain occupational health and safety issues had to be looked at, but cultural traditions were considered. With some resourcefulness, the hospital and maternity unit were able to accommodate the requests. Louise smiles. 'You'd never see anything like this in a hospital down south. It's truly amazing and such a learning experience for us all to watch women working in different ways.'

The situation was again different at a birth that happened a few days after this educational event. A healthy young Indigenous woman gave birth to her baby after an uneventful labour, but what followed wasn't uneventful: a massive

3.5-litre post-birth haemorrhage, sever anaemia, a trip to the operating theatre, intubation and ultimate transfer via CareFlight to a tertiary referral hospital.

Life in Louise's little remote hospital is never dull, and the staff are always kept on their toes.

Louise has discovered so much about caring for the birthing Yolngu women and their families. She's sat down with women while they are in early labour and been taught how to make necklaces by threading tiny shells and seeds onto fishing line. She's developed relationships with women over the course of their pregnancies and those women then seem to wait for her to come onto shift to start labour, so she can look after them while they birth their baby. She's been with one woman for four of her five births, another woman for three, and countless women for two. She's watched women instinctively breastfeed their babies without help or any sort of assistance – 'Women breastfeed here because that's what women do, without question.' She's developed lasting bonds and connections through telling stories and rubbing backs and has helped women get through the frightening sound of thunder and torrential rain if that is their phobia. She's listened to stories about living on country, stories of domestic violence and the incredible strength required to deal with it, stories about hunting, gathering and preparing food, stories about the love of weaving baskets and other women's work. She's learnt about the importance of promised marriages and keeping strong bloodlines by marrying the right skin, and she tries to understand the complexities of kinship law. She's listened to songline stories that are interwoven with the land, ocean and stars and seen the connection the women have with country and the strength that is gained from this. Oh, how she loves to be with these women. 'Where else are you privileged enough to be present for a traditional smoking ceremony of mother and baby?'

Louise has been present for beautiful quiet births, where beads of perspiration on the woman's upper lip are the only sign that birth is close, and where she's listened to women call in their traditional Yolngu Matha for the spirits of other women to come and help them. She's been present for births where there has been so much laughter and gaiety that she felt like she was at a rock concert – even a birth with a pregnant woman impersonating Michael Jackson and singing while her friend was in second stage and the other ten people in the room were rolling on the floor with laughter.

She's learnt that an OP labour (where the baby is lying in an occipito posterior position, with its spine against the mother's spine, which often causes back pain in labour) is quite normal and that the woman doesn't necessarily need an epidural – she just needs her midwife to stay with her. She's rediscovered that women are strong and beautiful creatures who can overcome incredible hardship, trauma, poverty and adversity and still not complain. She has truly learnt the value of holistic care for the mother and her family, and that just being with a woman is often enough. One of her most important lessons was to wipe away tears as mothers weep silently for their homeland and family. They weep because they are unable to birth on country, and because they have been separated from all that makes them whole.

Some of these girls are as young as twelve or thirteen but birth their babies with the strength and power of much older and more experienced women – putting their babies to the breast without hesitation, because this is what is expected and normal. She's watched these young girls become strong mothers who love and care for their babies with a resilience and maturity that she can't fathom.

There have been tiny, beautiful Indigenous babies born of women with chronic diseases, babies who are already battlers, who instinctively crawl to the breast from birth and remain there for the next week. In Louise's unit, so many of the babies are above their birthweight instead of weighing less by day three or five, because they never leave the proximity of the breast. Can you picture a baby who is twenty-four hours old already following her mother's movements and responding to her traditional language? These are the babies that Louise and her colleagues are privileged to watch grow and thrive under their care.

Louise feels as if these women were sent to teach midwives about normal birth and about the beauty and acceptance of being a woman. They exist to be mothers and grandmothers, and giving birth has nothing complicated about it – even if you suffer from a list of chronic diseases longer than your arm. Labour is part of the process that you experience in order to get your baby. All you need to help you through is the support and care of another woman – someone who rubs your back when you're in pain and lets you rest in between contractions. Nor is breastfeeding complicated – changes that are being seen now in maternity wards all over Australia, you just gently offer the breast and patiently wait for your baby to make the decision to feed. Yolngu women take their babies everywhere they go. You carry your baby on your hip and allow that baby or toddler to drink from the breast whenever they want. It's all very simple, and Louise finds herself encouraged by these beautiful women to 'keep it normal'.

Louise says, 'What an honour it is to walk alongside the Yolngu women and to hold their hand during the most precious of moments – sharing women's business. I just don't know if I could return to life down south! I've rediscovered my midwifery passion, and once again I'm feeling complete in my work. I feel like I've come full circle. I don't know what the next ten years will bring, but I'm looking forward to whatever comes my way.'

CHAPTER 14

Phone a PAL

Helen Cooke

Helen Cooke reminds you of your favourite blonde aunty. She has an infectious laugh and welcoming smile that belies her steadfast determination to keep mums and babies safe. Emergencies in maternity care do happen, and often with frightening speed. There are a lot of very lucky mothers and babies in Australia who can thank Helen Cooke for the fact that risk was recognised and dealt with quickly and competently. Helen's take-home message is safety in maternity care.

Helen is dedicated in her support of the Advanced Life Support in Obstetrics (ALSO) course, and has spent more than sixty volunteer weekends over the last fourteen years as part of the team that helps doctors and midwives to practise those skills all over Australia. Her husband, who also has a good sense of humour, has attended many, too. That's a whole lot of hours waiting in airports when you want to get home, yet when Helen is home, she's still caring for the ALSO instructors.

Cookie is the person you phone if illness or a family crisis crops up and you have to pull out of instructing on a course. She'll sympathise, tell you to look after yourself, lift the guilt, and find someone to replace you so the course can continue smoothly. All in her own time. With around fifteen instructors for each course and ten courses all over Australia every year, that's a lot of last-minute phone calls as well.

And for those in NSW who can't attend an ALSO week-end, Helen and her colleague Professor Warwick Giles were responsible for the rollout of FONT (Fetal Welfare, Obstetric Emergency, Neonatal Resuscitation Training), a NSW Health initiative that targeted the 5500 maternity services clinicians across the state with the aim of developing their skills for acting in emergency situations. Helen prepared the consistent learning package, ensured equipment was supplied, and provided the initial training for the 250 trainers who would go on to upskill those 5500 doctors and midwives. This magnificent effort entailed a lot of responsibility to ensure maximum safety for mothers and babies.

'I've been volunteering for both ACM and ALSO for about fourteen years and always felt very blessed to be able to work in a profession I feel so strongly about.' Helen is on the executive committee for the Australian College of Midwives as the hardworking treasurer. She says, 'I do remember one morning when I was driving to work I had a realisation that being a midwife was more than my profession – it was also my hobby.'

Helen has worked as a midwife in one of Sydney's larger hospitals, with higher risk pregnancies. One of her favourite memories of clinical midwifery goes back thirteen years to when she was privileged to support Heather during her first pregnancy. Helen met Heather when she was about 24 weeks pregnant, as her pregnancy was complicated by a number of medical conditions. Heather's obstetrician thought she would benefit from some midwifery care and asked Helen to see her on a regular basis.

Heather was eighteen, unemployed and in a relatively new relationship with her boyfriend, Dave. Helen saw Heather and Dave nearly every week throughout her pregnancy and they got to know each other very well. At that time Heather was consuming about 8 litres of Coca-Cola each day and, not surprisingly, this was causing a lot of the problems in her pregnancy. They talked about strategies and tools Heather could use to cut this amount down, and other issues, and their rapport stayed strong as Heather's pregnancy progressed to a normal birth at about 35 weeks. Baby spent a few weeks withdrawing from caffeine and growing up in the special care nursery, but went home well.

When Heather was pregnant with her second baby she asked early on to see Helen, a person she trusted and who made her feel strong about herself, which gave Helen great pleasure. She provided all Heather's care for the pregnancy, and they were both so proud of the fact that Heather had given up the Coca-Cola. At 39 weeks' gestation Heather went into labour, and when Helen arrived the birthing room held about fifteen members of Heather and Dave's family. It gets pretty crowded in a birthing room when so many interested spectators are sharing the experience, but Heather was happy at about 4 centimetres dilated, and Helen knew she'd let her know if she wanted it otherwise. Heather's labour progressed nicely even with all the family watching over her until suddenly, Helen remembers with a smile, when Heather was about 8 centimetres dilated, she shouted at all the family, 'Get out of here now!' Helen held the door open, and they all left quickly. About fifteen minutes later Heather started to push, and her beautiful baby girl was born.

Helen was there for Heather's third pregnancy, too. 'For me, it was such an honour and a privilege to be able to support Heather through her growth from being a frightened, angry teenager to the beautiful young woman she became.' Today Heather and Helen are still in contact. Heather has a profession, and three very beautiful and talented children. Helen knows she helped Heather along the way. 'For me, seeing I've helped is the most wonderful part of midwifery: supporting women to grow as mothers.'

Heather's story illustrates Helen's passion for working towards having a health care system that provides every woman with access to a lead midwife who plays a significant role in the provision of information and support for that woman.

Helen often feels saddened by the ongoing struggle for midwifery to be predominantly seen as caring for a woman outside of illness, and so to be recognised as a profession in its own right, distinct from nursing. In no way does she downplay the value of nursing, but the professions are very different in application and approach. In midwifery it is the woman who is the lead decision maker – not something that would work in serious illness. Helen believes one of the greatest midwifery skills is to do nothing but offer support for women to achieve their desired birth experience.

When Helen was appointed as the manager of the ante-natal ward in her large hospital in Sydney she felt a huge responsibility for the safety and security of the women admitted for care who weren't well. This meant needing to know as much as she could about the management of complex pregnancies, and she spent a lot of time researching interventions. It was the late eighties, when huge advances in in-vitro fertilisation were happening, and her ward of twenty-eight beds was filled with women having twins, triplets and quads as a result of their IVF treatments. She remembers one room of two beds and seven babies. Many of these women were on bed rest to prevent premature labour, even though this long-held custom was not research-based. Hours and hours of research later, having found little evidence in the literature to demonstrate that bed rest made any difference, Helen fought for women to be allowed out of bed and to move freely around the ward. In her heart she knows these efforts were worthwhile and today compulsory bed rest is no longer considered an acceptable treatment to prevent premature labour.

There are times when a new commitment is a challenge, like when she first started to teach Advanced Life Support in

Obstetrics courses and it had been a few years since she'd been working with birthing women. To realise that she needed to teach a non-midwifery skill such as the use of forceps and vacuum to doctors as well as midwives was very challenging but midwives needed to learn to be able to recognise safe practice and be advocates for women if needed. It's an essential part of the course that everyone on the team, doctors and midwives, understand safe practice and when to move on to another strategy if something isn't working. 'I found that the people at ALSO courses are very open to sharing the learning experience and sometimes you just have to give it a go. It becomes easier to teach as your confidence builds.'

It was the same when Helen began her position as the FONT project officer and took on the responsibility of coordinating and teaching FONT development to the new trainers who would carry the message across NSW from the city to the bush. It seemed a huge task to develop a statewide educational program for midwives and medical officers that covered both fetal welfare assessment and maternity emergency management. Research has shown that since the introduction of mandatory attendance at FONT courses for doctors and midwives in NSW there has been a reduction in babies and mothers with injury or worse from misdiagnosis and delayed treatment of problems in labour. Huge kudos to Helen and the FONT team.

Helen's work now takes her away from direct clinical care, and more towards a role that supports other midwives across NSW to work with women, though she does work clinically as a midwife with the state's perinatal advice line (PAL). This is a twenty-four seven phone line for clinicians (especially those in rural health centres and hospitals that only cater for low-risk mothers) to ring for clinical advice on the transfer of women across the state for higher level maternity care.

Helen finds her work fulfilling because it's different every day, though she's sad little of it involves contact with pregnant women. Her job ranges from the development of postgraduate face-to-face and online education for fetal welfare and maternity emergency management to clinical policy and guideline development for the state, and she coordinates the management of the clinical maternity database for NSW. She also works with local health districts throughout the state on the development of midwifery care models and service redesign, and takes part in clinical case review and risk management. It's a quietly achieving job that keeps making birth safer for women.

The fun part of Helen's day is when she's on the perinatal advice line providing support for the transfer of women who require a higher level of care or access to a neonatal intensive-care unit.

One of Helen's first calls when she began to work for PAL came in the middle of a freezing July night, the least inviting time to be out of bed. The call came from a very small town in western NSW, from a local GP not comfortable with birthing women and with no midwives on duty. He had a woman contracting in possible early labour eight weeks before her due date, and he was worried she'd begin to labour seriously.

It was her eleventh baby. He tried the nearest large hospital, in Dubbo, rang the paediatrican, the obstetrician and the RFDS . . . and that's when the fog came down like a blanket across the state, preventing an aircraft from either taking off from Sydney or landing in Dubbo. This GP was pulling his thinning hair out; he had a 32-week baby threatening to arrive who would probably require major resuscitation, no paediatric or obstetric support, and by now it was one in the morning.

So he rang the PAL line, and that night it fell to Helen to troubleshoot and coordinate resources from all over the state until a solution was found.

The main problem was that the RFDS aircraft could take off in the fog from Dubbo, but it would be too dangerous to land there again. Sydney was also fogged in. Finally it was decided that an RFDS midwife from Dubbo would fly to the small town where they could at least land, and stay with the mother and doctor, support the birth and resuscitation of the baby as necessary, then plan ongoing care.

They would have to manage as best they could until the fog cleared and transfer could be arranged. Which is what they did, and the mum, thankfully still pregnant, was flown out to Dubbo the next morning with the RFDS midwife. Mum's labour settled after she was treated, and after staying thirty-six hours in Dubbo she went home to her small town, where all went well with her baby's birth six weeks later.

PAL calls are all very different from one another. Some are as simple as organising a bed for a mum; others are as complex as organising transfer of a mother in premature labour who is

8 centimetres dilated, or a woman with escalating pre-eclampsia (high blood pressure that can lead to fitting) to a higher level of service. Helen believes the service offers an opportunity for the doctor or midwife at the other end of the phone to take a breath and sound out their options. Helen's experience and understanding of what is available means she can offer alternatives that may not have been considered. Even though she rarely meets the birthing woman personally, she follows her journey the following day.

Being the calm voice on the phone talking to clinicians anxious for best outcomes for their patients is complex and challenging, and adds another dimension to the care of women. Being able to offer advice and know she's helped women stay as close as possible to home and achieve a safe birth provides Helen with immense satisfaction. Her colleagues regard her as a beautiful midwife and friend, and through the perinatal advice line, others share that sentiment statewide.

CHAPTER 15

Birth at Home

Shea Caplice

There's a poster on the wall outside many birthing suites show-ing an ecstatic mother with her blinking, vernix-covered baby, fresh from a waterbirth, and in the background, the serene, smiling face of her midwife. You can tell this mother feels like she's just conquered the world. The smiling midwife is Shea Caplice.

Shea spent many years of her career as a homebirth mid-wife, and to this day when she goes to a birth she repeats a mantra to herself as she's driving: *Trust in the process.* Midwifery is exactly that. 'There's no typical week with this work. Pregnancy care takes up a lot of time, but you can be called out to a birth at any moment – and you never know what you're going to be called to or what you'll be called away from. You just have to drop everything and go.'

Shea works *with* women, alongside them, facilitating their journey through pregnancy, birth and into parenting. She has a gift for connecting with people and this, of course, enhances her work. As a homebirth midwife she sees the same woman throughout the pregnancy, labour, birth and afterwards, which means she builds a relationship with the mother and her significant others. For the better part of a year Shea is in their lives, and more often than not a strong friendship develops.

She acknowledges that when attending a woman in labour at the hospital whom she has not met before, the relationship has to be built instantly. 'I told someone the other day that I sell trust. By increasing trust we can reduce fear, and this has been the central tenet of my work as a midwife for many, many years.' So for Shea, as for most midwives, connection is paramount, as is finding common ground so that the woman can feel safe, trust her caregiver, relax and go with the flow. Shea uses the analogy of concentric circles when she explains her role at a birth, with the woman in the centre surrounded by her significant others, and Shea protecting the outer circle and coming in and out as needed.

Shea graduated in 1985 or thereabouts . . . it's too long ago to remember exact dates. During that era, the hardest thing for her was seeing unnecessary intervention in birth and routine care that disregarded the woman's individual needs. It was often more about the organisation than the woman herself. She found it challenging to follow policies she didn't believe in, and soon acquired a reputation for being outspoken. One of Shea's strengths is being an advocate for women and their families. She believes that's why she chose to work in home-birth, birth centres and now Aboriginal health. Working in these areas allows more autonomy and flexibility in her work as a midwife and a philosophy that is more woman-centred. 'That's the way I work best.'

Midwifery became Shea's passion. 'I feel I have both gained and given so much in my profession, and I wouldn't change a thing.' She says this tranquilly, and it reminds me of her earlier comment that to portray a calm confidence even when you are not feeling it inside is an important quality to have as a midwife.

She remembers a school friend who was the first of her peers to fall pregnant around the time Shea was training to be a midwife, and who chose to have a homebirth. While Shea wasn't present at the birth, her friend's story touched her deeply, particularly the fact that her friend was in control of the birth process and had a relationship with just one midwife throughout her pregnancy. This struck Shea as being so special that she approached a homebirth midwife to be her apprentice and attended homebirths with her for twelve months. That experience was pivotal, and homebirth became the cradle of learning for Shea. She learnt to work within the full scope of practice of a midwife, and many of the births she has attended fill her memory with images she can barely describe – 'loving events beautifully etched in my mind' – even if sometimes the outcome was not as expected. Shea's experiencev have also taken her in a creative direction. She has used her vision of birth and images that have resonated with her in the production of several iconic articles, videos and DVDs featuring natural birth and the philosophy of midwifery (links to view these can be followed from her website, sheacaplice.com).

Shea has always worked within the public health system in addition to practising privately because of her belief that women should be able to access good midwifery care no matter where they choose to give birth and whatever their income. However, working in hospital delivery wards has been challenging for Shea and remains so today. 'Too much machinery that goes *ping*, and too much dehumanising of a very important life event.' Shea acknowledges that the sheer number of women birthing in some big hospitals creates an environment of intervention and fear.

She also finds the shiftwork a challenge in the hospital, particularly night shift when the birthing business continues non-stop. In her homebirth practice Shea usually gets at least a few hours of sleep before being called up for those early morning babies, which she prefers to staying awake all night. Being on call for homebirths is a challenge, of course, as you inevitably miss out on important family, life and social events, but working with her midwifery partner Sheryl makes that so much easier. They've supported each other in caring for women and laughed and cried together through many long labour hours.

Midwifery, being predominantly women's business, is very political. It involves a high degree of advocacy for women and their families that may be against the hospital protocols and status quo. Also, as a profession that is predominantly

female it involves the inevitable power struggles and feminist challenges. 'I think that came as a surprise,' Shea says, 'as
was the actual personal growth you go through yourself when
attending so many life-changing events. It's a metamorphosis
of sorts; you discover so much about yourself. I'm incredibly
sensitive and intuitive, which is both a blessing and a curse.
Being with women when a baby dies is particularly hard, and
working with the Aboriginal community who have been disadvantaged for so long evokes a lot of feelings.' As a mentor
once told Shea, 'You can choose the silk instead of the sandpaper, but if you choose the silk you'll never get to the deeper
level,' and it's in those challenging moments that the connection and learning is most profound. To be with a woman who
has lost a baby you have to be prepared to walk into their pain
and be truly present. 'So I had to learn about self-care in order
to sustain the level of giving that is required. To fill the cup so
to speak which I don't think the health profession generally
does very well.

'I fortified my skills by attending homebirths, and this has
increased my confidence when working in hospitals. I never
felt concerned in hospital after doing homebirths on my own,
because there was always people around to help or to confer with. In attending homebirths I really learnt about what's
normal, so that when something's abnormal it's much easier
to detect.'

Shea often says to women, 'If you've never had anything
really challenging in your life, then labour and birth may be
it.' It's challenging, 'grassroots raw-edge life stuff' and she

feels privileged to witness that. With nurturing, kindness, trust and connection, Shea knows women will come through.

Both in and out of hospital, Shea's met a lot of kind, passionate midwives who work with women to facilitate empowering birth experiences. Some of them were her teachers, some her peers and others just chance meetings when working a shift together. She's grateful for them all, and for the wisdom that they have shared. 'It's a wonderful sisterhood.' But there have been men too – a number of wonderful male obstetricians were key in her midwifery education. These doctors, proponents for normal birth, stuck their necks out from their conservative peer group to back her up when a planned homebirth ended up in hospital. The ideology that they all had in common was aligned with the popular medical mantra of *First, do no harm*. They did not treat the woman as a number, or blindly adhere to protocols without acknowledging the woman as an individual, with her own set of needs and wants. Great, great men.

Having attended so many homebirths, does one stand out in Shea's memory? 'Probably the most pivotal was the first homebirth I attended on my own, which was by accident. I received a phone call one night from an expectant father who lived nearby saying that his wife was in labour and they were planning a homebirth, but they were unable to contact their midwife. He asked whether I would come and sit with them until their midwife arrived. I explained that I didn't have all the equipment, but he pleaded with me to come just until they could contact their midwife; if the birth was impending before she arrived, they'd go to hospital. So armed with a pinnard to listen to the baby's heartbeat, and a watch, I set off in the dark full of adrenalin.

'After I arrived, I soon realised that the woman was about to give birth and there was no time for her to go anywhere. Their midwife had been tracked down, but she was still on her way from the other side of the city. I went into midwife mode and reassured the woman that all was okay, and within half an hour of my arrival the baby was born. It showed me how normal birth really is, and that by keeping the birth environment calm and relaxed, minimising interruption or hindrance, the process will more than likely follow its natural course. I headed home at dawn, and it was the first of many drives home after a homebirth feeling elated and satisfied that I'd indeed found my passion.'

In regards to her own child's birth, Shea thinks midwives often do it hard. She was a midwife before she had her son, Lincoln, and she was always going to have a homebirth. She didn't trust the hospital system to allow her to birth under her own steam, nor to allow her partner to be involved, so she chose a midwife who was also her close friend, plus the midwife she was apprenticed to, to attend her birth. 'I think on some level just because I was a midwife and knew so much about the process I thought I would be able to give birth easily at home, but it was more challenging than I expected. The labour was very long, but I never felt that I couldn't do it or that I needed to go to hospital, and my beautiful 4.5-kilo boy was born at home.' It was a great experience, and provided her with an incredible insight into what birthing women go through. Even now Shea has a distinct memory of the effort it took to push Lincoln out. 'Becoming a mother was a great leveller for me. I think I just needed to pretend I wasn't a midwife and it would have been better for me, I just needed to get out of my midwifery head and let my body do it.'

Shea balanced the homebirth practice with working part-time in the hospital for over twenty years, but nowadays she's wound down the homebirths to focus her expertise on facilitating midwifery education and, most recently, supporting Aboriginal families. She's all too aware that Aboriginal babies die at double the rate of non-Aboriginal babies, so this is where she feels her skills are best utilised now.

In 2006 Shea was asked to set up a service out of the Royal Hospital for Women, Sydney, to care for Aboriginal and Torres Strait Islander families during pregnancy, labour and birth. Her team remains largely unchanged today. Shea works with a dedicated group of four midwives, an Aboriginal health worker, a social worker and a child and family health nurse. The service has won a number of awards for its innovation in maternal and infant health care for the Aboriginal community. Its cultural component, led by the service's Aboriginal health worker, is pivotal to this success. 'Women coming through the service have the cultural connection through the Aboriginal health worker, then get to know everyone during the pregnancy, so once they come into the hospital there's a familiar face with them. I feel privileged to be working with the traditional owners and first people of this country.'

Shea has even cisited the tiny hospital where I work to help educate our midwives on waterbirth. She's known as one of the experts on the subject, having produced an educational film on birthing in water called *The Art of Birth* and co-authored a chapter on waterbirth in a midwifery textbook. 'I saw a home waterbirth, and it just seemed so amazing and the woman was so relaxed that I became interested in the practice and decided to make a film about it.' *The Art of Birth* has been used nationally to help teach midwives about waterbirth, and in Shea's homebirth practice over 50 per cent of babies were born in water. 'Women are more comfortable and more able to feel in control in water.' Shea has witnessed many women who were so in control in water that they felt relaxed enough to reach down with their own hands and guide their baby out into the world. 'That is wonderful to see.'

For Shea, the use of water has always been a simple strategy for when the labour gets tough, as a natural form of pain relief. Often the women were so comfortable in the water Shea says they just didn't want to get out. Convincing the medical world of the benefits of water during labour and birth has been a challenge, but after many years of lecturing around the country Shea feels that it's now becoming more accepted.

Shea remembers being called to a birth on a cold, stormy winter's night. She was greeted by a blazing fire in the lounge room, the wading pool being filled by the woman's husband,

and the woman asking Shea to wake the other children. The mother climbed into the pool and quietly and peacefully gave birth, with five pairs of wide eyes gazing in wonderment. That was a magical and beautiful family moment for the sleepy children involved in the event. Shea says that she would definitely have had a waterbirth herself if it had been around when she gave birth.

When looking back on her midwifery career, Shea says the first images that surface are of the beautiful expressions of joy and wonderment on the faces of those present at the birth; in the faces of the parents, when meeting their baby for the first time, no matter what the birth has been like. 'There are few times in our lives when we come together in such a connected way – marriage, death and birth. I have been so grateful to be involved in such a significant life event with so many.' Shea hopes that even as she ages she will be able to attend births, perhaps as the wise woman sitting in the corner knitting!

The black-and-white photograph that adorns many delivery suite walls was taken for the archives of the NSW branch of the Australian College of Midwives in celebration of the midwifery profession. Shea had organised a photographer to come to the hospital that day to take photos of midwives in their work environment. The woman in the poster came into the birth centre in very strong labour, and birth was imminent. Shea quickly ran the bath and made her comfortable, but when she said she was going to get another midwife the woman began to push and asked Shea not to leave her. The baby was born quickly and Shea stayed and assisted, and the woman kindly consented to the photographer's presence. It was a one-in-a-million moment that was beautifully captured. The elation on the woman's face and the humble satisfaction on Shea's illustrates the art and miracle of birth.

CHAPTER 16

High-risk pregnancy

Kate Dyer

'Welcome to Maternal-Fetal Medicine, we are so sorry to tell you that your baby has . . .'

Kate Dyer has carried a camera in her bag every day for the last twenty-five years. Kate is almost always on call for high-risk pregnancies, and she never knows when a baby is going to arrive – and sometimes leave before the parents have had a chance to be parents.

Kate works with mothers and babies. Occasionally the mother's life is in danger; sometimes the babies die as soon as they leave their mother's womb; other babies live for a few precious days. Some will survive, but have lasting disabilities. And some will struggle in the beginning but grow up strong and perfect. Kate is there, holding hands with the parents and helping to steer the ship of grieving souls to a gentle harbour.

Kate is the clinical midwife consultant for high-risk pregnancy at the Royal Hospital for Women, Sydney. She's a godmother to three, and an honorary aunty to dozens of children and to hundreds of babies who have left this life. She is in awe of the families she works with because they have to make incredibly hard decisions, the type of decisions that will sometimes scar them for life. Kate has many scars herself, but she eases the pain by knitting tiny beanies and raggedy bears with 'bucketloads of personality' for parents to keep. These keepsakes carry the scent of their baby when the time comes for parents to go home with empty arms.

Kate can be boisterous, and has a wicked, irreverent sense of humour – she needs it for grounding herself – and a seemingly bottomless well of compassion. In 2014, she was awarded an Order of Australia for 'significant service to maternal-fetal medicine through clinical midwifery roles, and to the coordination of pre and postnatal care programs' as well as her dedication to families in times of need. She isn't keen to talk about herself, though, so unearthing this fact required some digging.

Kate became a registered nurse in 1978, and, surprised by how much she enjoyed the challenge, she studied to become a midwife in 1981 as well. After more study she was appointed as a clinical midwife consultant in 1988, and she's been working with high-risk pregnancies ever since. Despite being the technology queen, Kate has the skills to avoid the overuse of equipment to the disadvantage of the mother's labouring space.

Kate provides continuity of care; following the diagnosis of a baby with an abnormality, or of a maternal condition that places the mother and baby at risk, Kate is the midwife that some women will see every visit during their pregnancy. She inhabits the space where questions are answered, fears spoken of, and connection occurs between maternal-fetal medicine team members and the parents. She is one stable person throughout the woman's often-complex journey up until and after the birth.

When parents have a choice between interrupting a pregnancy and grieving now, or watching their baby grow with no prospect of a future and grieving then, most of us, parents, midwives, society in general, have no idea what to say.

Kate says, 'There can be the arguments about "Do we give the baby a life and, if so, what does that life mean?" Parents always hope for the perfect pregnancy and beautiful babies. Sometimes it doesn't happen like that.'

An abnormality that's incompatible with life and the decision to continue the pregnancy is a dilemma Kate has faced with parents many times – sometimes more than once with the same parents.

Kate sees her role as helping to create the story for that precious child, a story that will provide something tangible for grieving parents to hold on to when they leave the hospital. Hand and foot prints, strands of baby hair, the skilled and empathetic use of Kate's ever-present camera for a photo of a pale, tiny hand curled around a father's finger, or a tiny foot lying on a mother's palm; family portraits that can never be repeated. Along with details of birth, and weight and length, the story can include visitors, the staff involved, baptism and even the weather and world events from that day. And tiny hats and bears knitted by Kate.

A discussion with parents about an abnormality confirmed on ultrasound is a tough assignment. 'It's tougher for the parents. Sometimes we have to meet again tomorrow, or the next day, so that information can sink in, questions can be formed, options repeated. But the parents are still parents. Their baby might not stay, but that doesn't make baby less lovable or less precious than any other baby.' Parents need the right information in a timely manner, and providing nurturing pockets of silence to allow them to think is paramount.

Most midwives care for 'normal' women and healthy 'normal' babies, with all the joy, excitement, choices and hope this entails. The majority of the women Kate meets in her practice have just been told or are trying to get their head around the fact that there is a problem for their baby, or sometimes for themselves. For many of these women, they now need to grapple with often highly technical and complex information and decisions. Plus there is overwhelming shock, despair and grief at the sudden loss of the 'normal' baby they'd dreamed of. They're facing a future that is at best a child requiring increased medical input, and at worst lifelong challenges, a shortened life expectancy, or death. Caring for these families is not a career for the faint-hearted.

All Kate's midwifery is based on trying to find what is important for the woman and her family when things are bleak and getting bleaker. Together, they consider the choices and paint pictures of what the different decisions and scenarios might look like for the family. Will our baby survive, will our baby ultimately lead a normal life, how will we manage? Personalising care is imperative; Kate's focus is on *this* family and how her team can best support them. She spends hours every day talking with families about their baby's problem, helping them understand the technical and medical speak, reminding them of the joy and beauty in their baby regardless. She goes through a lot of boxes of tissues in her work.

Kate's role also entails a large amount of coordination, communication and negotiation, setting up the range of different specialists the woman will need to meet: baby surgeons, neonatal specialists, genetic specialists, maternal-fetal medicine specialists, social workers, and more. Trying to coordinate the consults to occur in one place over several hours so that the woman isn't travelling to all the different appointments can be a time-consuming challenge, but Kate's passion and that of those she works with means it usually all falls into a reasonable schedule for the mother. And then there is the coordination around the birth – who needs to be there, who needs to know about it, what specialists will need to be available and onsite or even in the birth space. Sometimes Kate thinks it's like planning a major event and then she remembers it *is* a major event – it's someone's birthday, and this baby's and family's future may depend on everyone getting it right at that moment. Somehow all of a sudden the phone calls, emails and discussions late in the evening are not a bother.

Because Kate is fortunate enough to be able to provide continuity of care to these women, she and her colleagues also try to find and maximise the beauty of a particular pregnancy at each visit. 'Sometimes this can be a challenge,' she says in one of her masterful understatements; she spends a lot of time thinking about where the beauty is for this family. If their baby will not survive, or will require lots of intensive-care support, how can she help them to come out the other side with memories of their loved and beautiful newborn, yet not be filled with overwhelming sadness and emptiness every day?

Over the years Kate has developed a toolkit, mostly thanks to the mothers who so graciously tell her what worked and what didn't work for them. She knits her small teddy bears, created with an even mix of love and hope, hats and soft blankets to give to the parents prior to birth. Her hope is that among all the equipment and technology of a neonatal intensive-care unit there is something familiar with their baby that has their scent all over it, conveying their love in the silence of loss. She never thought that one of her most important tools as a midwife would be her camera, but whenever possible she takes photos of the birth and the early newborn time. Birth for the women in Kate's care is usually heavy with medical equipment and exhaustion, and naturally it's hard for women to remember exactly what happened with all that is going on. Photos do help. They're also a little something to hang on to when your baby is in intensive care and you can't be with them at that moment. For parents enduring loss, photos are often the only proof that they're a mum or dad.

Kate gets to spend time with these women doing all the normal 'antenatal visit stuff', along with providing education about what to expect during labour and birth, regardless of how baby may be born. She loves this part of her role: a chance to simply talk about what is happening and to see a woman move from overwhelming devastation to planning the birth and welcome for her baby. More tissues.

Kate's role also means that for many of these women she'll be part of their birth, present when they meet their baby. For the mothers, this time is a combination of excitement, anxiety, exhaustion and relief mixed with a little fear but mostly hope, hope that the baby will breathe or that surgery will go well, or that someone got the diagnosis wrong. Sometimes Kate knows this mirrors how she feels – excited that the day has arrived, anxious for this family, exhausted from ensuring all is in place around them, afraid that things may go badly, but mostly hopeful that their baby will do well; hopeful that whatever happens this family has the strength, skills and resilience to come out the other side, changed but stronger.

Many women bring their baby or child back for an unannounced visit, which is one of Kate's greatest joys as a midwife, interrupting 'real work' to reflect and marvel at how well this child is doing. Seeing these families grow and blossom despite the challenges is a reminder of the resilience of families, the strength of the relationship maternal-fetal medicine midwives can develop through this work, and evidence that what they do matters. It makes Kate try even harder the next day, and definitely puts a warm glow in her heart.

Kate sees her midwifery role and that of the amazing team of clinicians she works with as a strong thread that is woven through each family's patchwork, the constant thread of their medical and midwifery interactions changing colours and helping to stop things from unravelling.

'I don't think at the beginning of my midwifery career I had any idea that I would end up working with women for whom things were not normal, or that care for this group of women would become my priority,' Kate says. However, over time she became aware that for women with complex pregnancies, particularly those with a fetal anomaly or experiencing perinatal loss, there wasn't much midwifery input in their care, and little choice offered or discussed. There was a lot of medical input, but hardly any continuity-of-care midwifery or care coordination. Kate's real light-bulb moment was when she started work at Westmead Hospital in Sydney in 1985 as the clinical midwife specialist caring for women with complex pregnancies and teaching fetal heart rate monitoring. 'I guess for me it just seemed right that midwives should be directly involved in the clinical decision-making and coordination of care for this group of women.'

She credits her greatest leaps in experience to spending hours with women during antenatal discussions, labour and the weeks following the birth, learning from them, listening to what they say and seeing how they respond to the different situations they need to face. Kate takes great pleasure in the many cards she has received over the years, with messages thoughtfully written by families letting her know what worked for them and, most importantly, why. She marvels at how these families found the time and energy to put into words their heartfelt thoughts following a time of great challenge and turmoil, and draws on these often as a reminder of what helps and why the work she does is so very important. 'While we can't always make things better, we can always work to do things better, so my cards are my treasure chest. They are also a place I go to when I'm feeling overwhelmed with the day or week. I open the treasure chest and read, and all of a sudden I'm reminded that for these families I did make a difference.'

Kate says the biggest gift she's been given by medical colleagues over the years has been the permission and freedom to develop the role of a midwife providing support for women with highly complex pregnancies. She's deeply appreciative of the faith, trust, respect and recognition that midwifery care for these women is as important and integral to good outcomes as high-tech obstetric care. It's impossible to list names and to do justice to all of those who have helped. Midwifery leaders and visionaries Pat Brodie and Nicky Leap have both played a significant role in Kate's early midwifery career and continue to inspire her in practice. Colleagues like Helen Cooke, a beautiful midwife and friend, have shown Kate over many years that following your midwifery heart over your head does work most of the time, and that given the right support and discussion your colleagues will come with you for the ride and ultimately enjoy it. Kate believes Dr Daniel Challis has been an important part of her midwifery career – his vision for setting up a midwifery-led and coordinated maternal-fetal medicine (MFM) department changed the face of care for this group of mothers in her hospital. Over time the service has evolved to include a specific MFM midwifery group practice, a team of fantastic midwives dedicated to making sure every woman 'feels like the most important woman in our world at that moment'.

One of the challenges and joys of Kate's midwifery role is that no day or week is the same and no amount of planning will make things predictable. She has learnt that there's no reason to worry about this, because somehow it all works out.

Every day they have MFM clinics, which bring in a mix of women they've met before and new women for whom a diagnosis awaits. A typical day involves looking at the schedule, identifying who they're seeing and what will need to be or has already been arranged for them, which specialists are coming to provide consultation, who needs a tour through the NICU (neonatal intensive-care unit), an antenatal visit, a genetics consult, a lengthy discussion about the potential outcomes for a baby. And what babies are likely to arrive.

Today, Kate's first consult is a woman at 19 weeks' gestation. She was told two days ago that her baby's bowels are outside of its body, a condition called gastroschisis. This is her first appointment with Kate, and although they've spoken via phone to make the appointment and discuss the baby's problem, she is naturally very scared. She's done some reading on Dr Google, and this has not helped her anxiety.

An ultrasound scan confirms the gastroschisis. Following this, Kate's role is to again explore with the woman what this all means in non-medical speak. Kate shows her some pictures to convey the baby's problem, they talk at length about pregnancy care and what will happen for baby following birth. Mum sees pictures of other babies and children with the same problem. Kate takes a booking history in among their discussions and provides the twenty-four-hour contact number. This mum's baby will be born with the help of Kate's team, who will see her at each visit and be with her at birth; she is reassured that her baby is likely to do well, but the thought that her baby will go to surgery within hours of birth and be in intensive care for many weeks is overwhelming. Kate provides tissues and tea before the mother meets with the specialist baby surgeon who will ultimately fix her baby's belly. In the meantime, Kate sees the next woman.

The next woman is 18 weeks pregnant. She's been scanned and seen by the MFM specialist, who explains that there is twin-to-twin transfusion syndrome, a problem that can occur for identical twins where there is unequal sharing of blood between them. Laser of communicating vessels is recommended as a potential treatment. Once again, Kate's role is to discuss in plain English what all this may mean, and of course the mother is very teary after hearing that one or both of her twins may not survive. After a lengthy conversation with Kate, the couple decide to give their babies every chance possible and consent to the treatment. Kate arranges a hospital bed and organises the mother's admission, and secretly prays that this will all go well. At the same time she marvels at the expertise available in the MFM team that makes this treatment possible. 'Twin-to-twin transfusion is an awful complication. Without even thinking about it, I promise to pop up and see them later in the day.'

Meanwhile, the MFM team have just finished meeting with a family already known to Kate, and have given this family the news that their baby has a chromosomal anomaly not compatible with life outside of the uterus. Kate and the parents had known there were several structural anomalies, but finding that chromosomes are abnormal has really changed the picture. Kate is asked to meet with them, and she's overwhelmingly sad for this family. After much talking and thinking, they make the difficult decision to continue pregnancy and provide their baby girl with comfort care after birth. That means holding her, loving her, and losing her. Kate talks about what needs to be put in place for when that time comes, they name their baby, and Kate gives them a pink knitted teddy bear. They make an appointment to come back next week to meet a range of specialists to plan further.

Kate gets a call to say she has a visitor, so she excuses herself and pops into the waiting room to meet beautiful baby Archie and his mother, who are going home after a very challenging time – but not before saying a heartfelt thankyou to all of the team. Archie has had major chest surgery and spent a lot of time hooked up to some very impressive machinery in intensive care, and he is now perfect. Yep, this is one of Kate's greatest joys, and her eyes fill with tears as she hugs the mum.

The next woman has a baby with an abnormal heart who will ultimately do well. She has met the baby heart doctor, social worker and neonatal team, toured the NICU, and all is in place. Kate met this family at 18 weeks of pregnancy, and the mother is now 40 weeks and getting excited about meeting her baby. An induction is planned for tomorrow to allow all the right people to be available for baby's immediate care. Kate takes the mum's BP and feels her tummy; baby is a good size and well down in the pelvis. An internal examination shows the cervix is very ready for labour. They discuss any last-minute questions, and Kate is almost as excited as the woman about meeting her baby tomorrow.

Kate glances at the clock – it's 2 p.m. and the next lady is waiting to be seen. The phone rings and it's a new referral. She takes the details, woman's name, contact number and reason for referral.

The next woman's baby is tiny at 26 weeks of pregnancy, and is not growing. It's likely that baby will need to be born over the next few weeks. Kate talks with the mum about preterm birth, caesarean birth and preterm babies, and they plan to tour the NICU tomorrow. Kate gives the woman the first dose of steroids to help mature her baby's lungs. She monitors the baby's heart rate for a while, and they talk about getting prepared for baby's premature arrival. Kate provides tissues and a teddy bear and tiny hat for the baby when the time comes. The size of the little hat and bear reminds them both how fragile and exciting new life can be. They both rely on the hope that everything will be okay.

It's now 4 p.m. The phone rings, and it's one of the birthing suite midwives to let Kate know that one of the women she has been involved with has just given birth to her stillborn baby girl at 24 weeks. Kate refreshes her lipstick – the midwife should not look more exhausted than the mother – takes her camera, some canvas frames for footprints and a very deep breath. She has spent many hours with this family over the last week, as they made heartbreaking choices for their baby with multiple anomalies. They presented overnight with the baby not moving. Kate spoke with them several times in the early hours of the morning, and they knew she would come when needed.

Over the next hours Kate admires their beautiful tiny baby, helps them bathe and dress her, and takes photographs of them as a family, as parents. Kate photographs her little feet with her knitted teddy and a blanket made by her mum. They talk about what might have been, and Kate is relieved that the baby girl made her own choice and that this wasn't left to her parents. She talks with her midwifery colleagues about what else needs to be done. Paperwork, so much paperwork. Kate will see this family in the morning and give them the photos and CD of baby along with a memory book; it's something to hold on to in the weeks and months ahead, some tangible evidence that they really did have their gorgeous little girl.

Before she leaves she remembers to ring the new referral lady and give her an appointment for two days' time. On her office desk someone has placed a card. She opens it. It's a thankyou card from a family who gave birth last week, full of heartwarming and honest words of gratitude and appreciation. Just reading it brings her to tears; the timing is perfect. Kate places the card in a prime position on the bookshelf – later it will join the others in her treasure chest, a box full of wonderful and wise words from families.

She heads home, and after dinner she reviews the photos of the tiny girl and puts them on a CD. For a moment Kate's a mess of tears and dripping nose. She does use a lot of tissues in her work, but mostly she feels so very privileged and honoured to have been part of this family's journey, which really helps her to get up tomorrow and do it all again. She then makes a little book. 'I never thought when I entered midwifery that birth and death could be so closely linked.'

CHAPTER 17

Nurturing neighbours

Heather Gulliver

Across the bay from the soaring mass of Mount Tavurvur, the active volcano of Rabaul, Papua New Guinea, Heather Gulliver opens the curtains to the gentle dawn light.

It's been another night of restless sleep, with local alarms blaring from power interruptions and the guards in the security compound where Heather lives breaking into shouts and songs to join the chorus. Not a lot of shuddering of the earth lately – not many 'gurias', earthquakes, over the last month. Tavurvur hasn't vented for nearly a year now and the last town-destroying eruption was in 1994.

Heather sits with her laptop on her knees in her lounge/kitchen/office and mutters a thank you as the internet springs into decent life. She's finally able to source a professional practice guideline she's been waiting for and quickly emails it out

to all of the eleven other team members across the five different provinces in PNG before the web crawls to a halt. Then
she feels a sudden kick from the chair she's sitting in – was
that a little guria? The light hanging over the dining table is
gently swaying . . . probably only a two on her apartment
Richter scale.

She heads off to work in the intense, sticky heat, and the
smell of tropical foliage and dusty roads mixed with ash lines
every breath; it's the dry, windy season. When she arrives at her
shared office, four women on laptops are joined like spokes of
a wheel to Heather's surge protector in a tiny office meant for
one person. The deafening fingernails-on-chalkboard screech
of a buzz-saw tearing into the wall next door makes thinking
in a clear and logical way a little challenging.

Heather is working in the provinces of Papua New Guinea
as a clinical midwifery facilitator, as part of the Bachelor of
Midwifery program training PNG nurses as midwives in a
joint effort between the PNG and Australian governments.
She is helping PNG midwives to become educators in their
own right, and changes for the good are happening. Modern
midwifery and medical learning is being strengthened, simple
yet lifesaving strategies are being implemented, and – though
creakingly slowly because the infrastructure is still patchy – the
knowledge is being passed on to new and outreach PNG midwives by women from their own culture to improve the safety
of birthing women and their babies.

For Heather, the successful nurturing of a PNG midwife
lecturer comes with a swell of emotion. To see the development

of computer skills and the growth of confidence, the placing of a heading on a picture slide, is a thrill. Sitting at the back of the room watching a new lecturer share a simple hands-on manoeuvre that could control post-birth bleeding and save a woman's life, and the wonder on the faces of the rapt students, makes her want to clap.

Heather is an intensely spiritual woman who believes in helping mothers who suffer hardship and tragedy too often as a consequence of being a woman in PNG. Skill development for midwives is not readily available in PNG, particularly not for those serving in the rural areas, and avoidable maternal and neonatal death is far too common. So for the last four years Heather has been one of the midwifery educators sharing her knowledge while living in challenging conditions in different provinces of PNG. Her mentorship often leads her to work with birthing women or newborn babies in adverse conditions, or to be at the end of a crackling phone line supporting a graduate student midwife struggling to keep a mother alive in a remote health centre while awaiting transfer to a distant hospital. Heather and her peers are fostering courage among the new breed of PNG midwives to help them stand beside birthing women with compassion and offer protection, to be the safety net for these women and their babies – and then to share these concepts in front of a classroom of eager student midwives.

It all began in 1978 during Heather's final year of general nursing. Although untrained in midwifery, she was given the job of supporting a young single woman in preterm labour at about 26 weeks' gestation, whose baby was deemed unable to be saved because of prematurity. Heather says, 'In this era, away from metropolitan centres, this was happening all over because we didn't have the technology or neonatal intensive-care wards we have today.'

Heather recalls that this young labouring woman's unmarried status required her being called either 'that girl', in a demeaning tone, or 'Mrs' when in earshot of the public. To Heather it felt punitive. The other nurses were not so kind, and the young mother asked Heather to stay beside her when her baby came. Her little daughter slipped into the world lusty and rosy pink, and Heather helped her up to meet her mum briefly before the midwifery staff returned. Those few short minutes of shared connection between a young nurse and a grieving mother – their wonder at the astounding perfection of the tiny baby lying on her mother's warm skin – had a profound impact on Heather. This baby, Rose, was taken from her mother because it was thought better for all concerned, and it took many hours of isolation, tucked in a corner as if already passed, for her baby skin to become pale, her cry to weaken and for her to fade away. Thankfully nowadays a baby like Rose, if she could not be saved, would lie furled against her mother's skin until the passing.

From that day forward Heather couldn't call a pregnant, labouring or new mother 'that girl'. She wanted to see all new-born babies welcomed on their mother's bare chest, with her heartbeat the primary source of their connectedness. Heather looks upon all labours and births as sacred events – no matter when and where they take place.

She still has the small gift this young woman gave her when she was discharged home after her 'miscarriage'. The tiny vase has delicate painted pink and red roses on it and reminds Heather of those few hours they shared together, in which she learnt how simple kindness and suspension of judgement can open up a space for joy, and that every woman and new baby deserves their meeting to be surrounded by love, irrespective of the eventual outcome.

As with many other midwives, no doubt, there were obstacles to Heather becoming a midwife. Leaving a young family and glorious home and farm to study midwifery in the city challenged her own ideas about motherhood. This challenge has remained present throughout her work as a midwife, as she follows her path to champion women's rights in birth.

Heather says, 'I don't think I was clear about what I was expecting when I began my journey into midwifery. I continue to be confronted by factors that impact on women's rights to respectful care during their lives.

'Sometimes here in PNG, I feel like I'm cupping a low-burning candle against a strong wind in the darkness . . . when suddenly someone I'm mentoring seems to light up with a glorious moment of understanding a new knowledge or skill, or I witness protection for a woman or baby during a time of vulnerability, or sometimes I see a lifesaving activity.' These moments of joy make it all worthwhile for Heather.

Heather models and fosters self-reflection in midwifery practice. For her, the honesty and insight shared by her PNG counterparts demonstrates a courage and vision in the face of adversity that would seem impossible to many. When these stories are shared, often with pride, and definitely as a sign of greater knowledge or resilience, she knows being a midwife is still a song she loves to sing, currently in 'a choir of voices from PNG'.

Heather says it's difficult to understand how women in PNG can carry a burden of grief and loss with such calm and acceptance. Yet, just a few hours south in Australia, birth has become less and less of a natural life event and more an orchestrated intervention at a time someone other than the baby chooses.

Heather thinks that perhaps she did enter midwifery with an idealistic expectation of women around the world reclaiming their power when it came to birth, and maybe she has seen a lot more suffering than advancement in the status of women. But she continues to love the clinical work, even if it is definitely sweaty work with resource difficulties such as a lack of electricity and running water when the system fails. She's always drawn back to being present, respectful and joyful – how else could you be, at such a remarkable event in a woman's life? 'How fortunate am I,' Heather says, 'to be a midwife?'

Heather believes her success is due to her own many mentors over the course of her career, from Margaret Santo Spain, who helped Heather find her voice during her first few years in private practice, to 'the two Sues' – Kildea and Kruske, who still strive for improvement in Indigenous Australian health outcomes and to bring birthing back to the country.

She greatly admires Caroline Homer and Pat Brodie for their professional leadership over many of her years as a midwife; working with them now on a shared initiative is a fabulous outcome. Recently, she's also been working with a hugelu influential PNG midwife who speaks with a quiet voice and barely reaches Heather's shoulder. Ellie Natera has taught Heather that little women with big hearts can reach great heights and positively influence many lives, rolled around laughing when Heather displayed her frustrations in an exuberant fashion, and made her feel loved when she was a long way from home and family.

Another wise PNG midwife, Gwaidong, taught Heather a lot but also sought her counsel during complex cases, helping her to feel valued and that she was making a difference in her work with PNG women and babies. Heather's Madang midwifery adventures with Lois Barry will also remain warm memories.

But back to Mount Tavurvur, and a normal day for Heather in the town of Kokopo in the Rabaul district, PNG.

Internet – tick. Making it into the office – tick. Now to support the lead coordinator of the midwifery education program. There are twenty-two new student midwives in the eight-week lecture block who need to be placed in hospitals and clinics to gain clinical experience with mothers and babies. Heather is acutely aware they are drawing to the end of the agreement between the two countries and need to build the midwives' problem-solving strategies and learning skills as much as possible in the remaining time they share. The coordinator of the program is keen to have this supported teaching opportunity, and they lock in her leading at least one session every day during the theory block. Heather helps the coordinator choose one of the unit topics, and commits to finding some teaching resources on twins.

Then it's time for a session with the newest Papua New Guinean midwifery educator. She and Heather go through, slide by slide, the session on malaria in pregnancy that the educator has worked on for the last few days. They add prompts to guide her with student questioning, and the new educator speaks with pride about being able to 'add in text' to some of the slides and bring in slides from other resources Heather provided during their last session. Heather's excitement is a little noisy, so two of their PNG colleagues hear them celebrating this achievement, and Heather asks the educator if she can show them how it is done on one of their laptops. She watches as they gather together – standing room only, away from those power cords – and listens to the ooohhhs and aaahhhs as the empowered educator skilfully demonstrates for her colleagues with some basic PowerPoint presentation skills. Heather is quietly satisfied with the gain of another small way in which these committed young women can sustain the growth of PNG midwife training into the future.

The lead coordinator comes back, by which time Heather has found a few resources on twins. She shows the coordinator how to develop a title page and put her name on it – doing so feels both symbolic and like a milestone. At last they can work together to strengthen the coordinator's engagement with the theoretical component of the program, and they go on to discuss different interactive methods she could use to engage the students. She has some great ideas, and asks Heather to come in at the end of her session to answer any difficult questions the students have about twins. They decide this feels like a good partnership plan.

As the morning rolls on the noise of the building renovations continues to threaten the women's sanity. The timber and tile saws are working on the step outside the office, large timbers are being dropped on the floor above, sink benches are being hammered into the wall beside them, men are climbing past the window on scaffolding and hammering new guttering; the cacophony of different sounds bores into their brains. The decision from on high to renovate the office and teaching classrooms while they are in use was not finding favour.

The open-door office policy is great for fostering learning and engagement but does mean delays due to socialising. There's a visit from the head of school to say they'll be opening an unused ward in the hospital as a modified maternity ward. It's reassuring to know some of the 200 or more birthing women they serve each month will not be sent away to find transport to another hospital over half an hour away via a very rough road to have their babies. Being sent away impacts on entire families, who must travel to bring the birthing women food and water. Not so fortunate are the antenatal women, who won't have a service to use for some months.

The temporary closure means all the equipment and resources, including all the teaching material supplied by the initiative or donated by Heather, needs to be either packed up in the maternity ward for storage or moved to set up another labour, postnatal and nursery ward in the hospital. That will be a very big job for everyone.

The head of school also tells them that one of the Memorandum of Understandings (MOUs) has been returned from a second legal branch with some changes she would like Heather to look at. Signing of MOUs is essential for the students to be able to access the required clinical practice areas in different sites across different provinces, and Heather is extremely keen to complete the process, which has been ongoing for five months. It takes more than two hours, but it must be done.

Then Heather and her clinical midwifery facilitator (CMF) colleague drive up to the closed ward in the midday heat and begin emptying filing cabinets and gathering resources that need storage during the ward closure. They fill the seats and back of the car with books, obstetric models, a birth ball and the birthing chair Heather's husband made before driving back down to the school.

Heather just has time to make sure her teaching partner is happy with her session resources and to make a quick coffee before they head upstairs for her partner's teaching session on bleeding in pregnancy. She does exceptionally well considering her quiet demeanour and the renovating racket. They return to the office at 4.20 p.m. for a short debrief – students engaged well, asked questions, and with delight Heather senses her colleague's boost of confidence.

Heather's PNG colleagues go home, and she and her CMF colleague remain in the office to meet with an obstetrician to discuss several issues of their program work. He agrees to run a session for the students on manual vacuum aspiration, but reminds them to bring this equipment down from the ward before it gets packed up or lost in the move that starts tomorrow.

Heather then redrafts the day's teaching sessions, removing graphics to make them easier to print for the students, considering the shortage of ink in the printer. These versions are printed as master copies, and filed and uploaded onto the drive for her PNG counterpart and team to use for future programs.

Heather's CMF colleague returns after her evening meal break to run a session on computer skills for the students. The two Aussie midwives debrief about another interesting day before Heather drives up to the ward in the dark to find the equipment needed for the vacuum aspiration teaching session.

She spends some time with the Papua New Guinean lead clinical midwife discussing challenges related to the ward closure, lessons learnt from prior closures, and how they can work together around these. Heather agrees to find some bags to store resources in her home for safekeeping.

The doorbell rings and a labouring woman is admitted to the temporary labour ward. The PNG lead clinical midwife, who is four hours past her shift finish time, have to leave. It's after 8 p.m. Heather swings her full billum over her shoulder, then hears the midwife in the labour ward calling for her colleague by name with distress in her voice. She swings her bag off her shoulder, grabs a pair of gloves and joins the midwife, who has struggled to deliver a baby that was jammed by the shoulders. The baby is only gasping occasionally, and it is obvious it needs help to breathe.

The midwife wants to stay with the mother to help with the placenta as there is also a risk of postpartum bleeding, so Heather agrees to care for the baby, and shortly afterwards a nurse arrives to help with the neonatal resuscitation. Heather talks through each of the strategies she uses to help the baby breathe, and after a few minutes the baby is breathing well but needs some oxygen to remain a good colour. After reassuring the mother, they do a newborn examination and Heather talks the midwife and mother through the ongoing management of baby.

Heather checks with the midwife if she is happy for her to go home, and within half an hour she's back in her apartment and enjoying her longed-for shower. She wonders how it must have been for the new mother when she talked through what she was doing in that critical situation. She hopes she spoke with clarity and in a reassuring way, to both the mother and the staff she was working with. She is grateful for the chance to help a baby to breathe and to support a Papua New Guinean nurse by sharing this knowledge. Building bridges between new knowledge and bedside care remains a critical element in Heather's midwifery work. She wonders about progress with the ethical consent for her planned breech birth training. It could be so useful! She needs to stop thinking about work and listen to an ABC show so she can let another working day in PNG finish. For now.

CHAPTER 18

Baby whisperer

Michael Dixon

'Hello, I'm your midwife today.'

Michael Dixon's quiet voice is calm and definitely masculine. The woman's partner looks like he swallowed a canary at the unexpected announcement. 'Don't they call you a midhusband?'

Michael's heard it all before. He works as a midwife in my small hospital and is a down-to-earth shift worker with a gift for helping people find inner reserves. This anthology wouldn't be complete without at least one of the men of our profession sharing insight from a male perspective.

Michael says he was a callow and naive lad when he left the country to become a nurse in the big city, but I can't believe that because I've always found him to be quietly wise. Nicknamed Digger, because his birthday's on Anzac Day, or

Mikey D, as he's known by the midwives, he's a lovely guy. He leavens our feminine squabbles with an innate ability to see the good in people and with his disinterest in gossip. We love him. And more importantly, the birthing women and families love him too. They sense his faith in natural birth and draw strength from his presence in the corner of the room. You could walk into a birthing space and not notice Michael, unobtrusive, quietly spoken, yet fully aware of the needs of the birthing woman and her family.

Michael says he entered nursing with no burning ambition; a friend suggested it was a good career. Initially, he says, he had no idea what to do with his life. Nursing turned out to be a great decision, where he made good friends and learnt a bit about life, but he certainly didn't think that it would be the sum total of his contribution to society. As an aside, he's a darn good dad, too.

But it seems midwifery had plans for Michael. Fast forward four years from graduation and he and his 'strong and beautiful partner', heavy with child, moved down from their isolated farm to a large country town to take care of her parents' house for twelve months. Immersed in the coming birth, the parents-to-be had read all the birthing classics – Michel Odent, Grantly Dick-Read, Janet Balaskas and so on – and felt that the local hospital would not be able to help them in their journey to a peaceful, natural birth. This was 1985, so they were probably right – thankfully times have changed since then.

They engaged the local homebirthing midwife, Rhonda, who encouraged and supported the ideas that they had researched, and impressed them with her professionalism and gentle manner.

When Paddy decided it was time to make his way into the world, Rhonda was there to guide them on their journey to parenthood. Michael says, 'First babies always demand a trial of strength and character from their mothers. Jacky was up to the task. She had prepared physically, emotionally and spiritually for the birth. It was tough. Labouring all night, under the shower for hours, walking, stomping, resting, cursing, but mostly she dwelt in a subconscious primal state of being.'

Rhonda understood this state, and Michael watched and was careful not to break the trance. To Michael, the rapport between midwife and woman seemed based on a telepathic understanding. He was an observer and helper. Paddy was born a few hours after the sun rose, in their lounge room before an open fire. Michael had witnessed a calm and peaceful birth for the first time. 'I had become a father, but I'd also been witness to the sacred sanctity of birth. I felt at the time that birthing was the domain of women, something that was culturally and spiritually feminine. What place was there for a man in this environment?'

Yet two years later, he was enrolled in a midwifery education program at an outer Sydney hospital, though it was a career move rather than a calling. Fifty per cent of the mums had no English, and the district had over one hundred language groups. He said he became particularly good at sign language and visual clues. During the twelve months of intense training, he found that he was well received by staff and new mums alike.

Positive feedback and the 'warm and fuzzies' of the work encouraged him. Also, Jacky birthed their second child, Ella, this time in a hospital while he was on duty in the labour ward. By 1988, he was a registered midwife.

Michael worked for six months in his training hospital, gaining experience and confidence. In that time he managed labours and births, as well as antenatal and postnatal care, in the busy maternity unit. He particularly enjoyed working with unwell infants in the special care nursery, and his skills became a useful addition to the next hospital he worked in. It was time to move back to the bush.

They headed north up the coast of New South Wales again, and for a brief period Michael worked at a mid-sized base hospital for which a male midwife was an oddity. 'They were unsure of my notions of active birth, radical stuff at the time, but they appreciated my skills with sick babies. I never felt quite at home there.'

Michael and Jacky finally found their little piece of bush again, well out of town along miles of dirt road. Jacky was pregnant with their third child when they moved to their current location by a fickle creek crossing. Their home sits in a tiny valley, the creek at its feet, the trees all around, and the neighbours a long walk away from the house that Digger built.

They settled there twenty-five years ago now. The matron of the local hospital gave Michael a position in the maternity ward, where his midwifery found a home. Again, the fact that Michael was a male midwife had novelty value, but he quickly made friends with the young and older midwives, joined the local soccer team, and soaked in the tranquillity of the bush and his eclectic music at home. Daughter Nina was born at Michael's new hospital – another quick and natural birth.

Michael has been working with the local women, families, midwives and doctors ever since then, and he feels very much at home. As a male midwife he is fully accepted by the community and staff. He is one of the midwives who facilitatesthe evening antenatal classes for new parents, having so much to give to the dads as well as the mums, and is often the first face seen by new mothers-to-be as they book into the maternity unit for their coming antenatal visits. 'We've seen many great changes in maternity care in the time I've been here, and the philosophy of care is improving every year.'

He feels that the greatest asset of the maternity unit is community trust in and support for the staff and doctors. Because it is a small country hospital, the families have a sense of ownership of their maternity ward. The midwives, staff and doctors are all committed to the community, as they are members of the community too. Many of our kids and grandkids were born at the hospital, and some of the staff too. 'We work as a team, bringing our own strengths to the mix and complementing each other to create a sum greater than the parts.'

In this small-town unit, quite a few have come and gone, leaving their imprint, but many have worked here for most of their working lives and have difficulty imagining working elsewhere. 'We learn from each other and grow together as professionals and people and I hold my colleagues in the highest esteem.'

We get to practise many of our skills on a daily basis. Anything can happen on any shift. We offer antenatal and postnatal care. We manage labours, attend caesareans, and care for the newborn. We have a midwives' antenatal clinic and see antenatal outpatients. We help with mothercrafting and breastfeeding. We have recently been able to offer a birthing pool for labour and birth. But Michael thinks, most of all, we just sit and talk with our mums and families, and that's perhaps the most rewarding aspect of our vocation. It's the human interaction, sometimes funny and sometimes sad, but always personal.

Michael has become a participant in birth and parenting education over the past ten years. There are small groups of soon-to-be parents that gather for six evenings to share their stories, aspirations, hopes and fears, and Michael says he learns as much from them as they do from him. He's known for his emphasis on feelings and emotions, and the profoundly transformative nature of birth and parenthood. Of course he deals with the practicalities and discusses the not always foreseeable aspects of the journey, so that the group is aware of obstetric and neonatal realities. But his main purpose is to allay any fears and anxieties and promote confidence and positivity.

One area in his work that is perhaps unique is his involvement with dads. He often has discussions with new fathers about the joy and responsibilities of fatherhood. He admits he has no formal training in this area – just a broad range of experience and, he hopes, a little bit of wisdom. Dads can sometimes feel a bit peripheral in a maternity ward. Many dads take a while to find their role in the new world of parenting. His advice to them is to try to be supportive and caring for the new mum and their precious new baby. Michael is aware that sometimes men are not good at expressing their emotions and feelings about the transformation of their lives. It's not always an easy transition to the role, but luckily most take to fatherhood like ducks to water. It can be the moment boys become men.

When asked why he chose to become a midwife, Michael puts it like this: '"*Midwife*" is apparently an Old English word meaning "with wife (or woman)". This is my response when I'm called a "midhusband". "Midwife" is not gender specific. The role certainly is the province of women, and rightly so. It took a while for me to find my place in a world of oestrogen and oxytocin. I still have my doubts from time to time; every woman has a right to be cared for by another woman. I do understand if my presence has a negative impact or is not wanted. But, over the years, this has been an uncommon experience. I sometimes get called "doctor", but I soon set that straight. I think that just being myself, being empathetic and caring, skilful and professional, positive and appropriate, means I am accepted as someone who has a meaning and reason for being there.

'I think every birthing mum remembers their midwife. Having been with birthing women for twenty-five years in a small country town, people know me or know of me. That helps to break the ice. I have a good rapport with the local Indigenous community, respecting their culture and ways and enjoying a laugh. Sometimes I have more issues with dads than I do with the mums. C'est la vie; I'll do my best to win them over. I wish I could remember everyone I've been involved with, as they do remember me. Some births or some incidents are indelibly stamped in memory. Some people and some ante-natal groups really stand out. Times shared with colleagues are often precious; we laugh a lot, talk a lot and hug a lot. We're a pretty close-knit crew. Not every shift is easy. Some days are extremely challenging.

'This profession teaches you a lot about life. That's what it's all about, really. Every once in a while, we have to deal with very sad and tragic circumstances. These events can make it really difficult to come back to work the next day. Sometimes the sadness seems too much. We might blame ourselves for something that was out of our control. We might find a weakness in our confidence. We might have major disagreements with people we trust and respect. We might never get over it, or we might grow as a person and a professional. We might console our colleagues as much as our grieving families. The challenges of being a good midwife and a good person are inescapable and welcome.

'So how do I keep coming back to work every day? Good coffee is the right start. No, seriously, it's the sense of worth. The inspiration of humble people. The sense of being involved in something intrinsically good. The respect for nature and sci-ence. The respect I have for myself and humanity. The laughs and the love. Really, just the humanness of what happens in a maternity unit.

'What have I learnt along the journey? You can't be right all the time, but you do your best. Whatever you give, you get back in multiples. That new mothers shine a beautiful light in a sometimes dim world. Babies are our teachers. Fathers are strong. Midwives are some of the best people in the universe. We are there to guide and protect a social and biological transition to the next generation. We want to help that transition to be the most empowering, safe and joyful event that we can, and I believe that we make the world a better place. Love and peace to all the midwives in the world.'

CHAPTER 19

From midwife to mother

Devon Plumley

Devon Plumley had been a midwife for a long time before she fell in love, had her fairytale wedding, and gave birth to her first baby. This is Devon's story about being a mum, about all that advice she gave to women over the years – which she wouldn't change, but gained a new understanding of – and what she's doing now. I really wanted to know how Devon felt being a first-time mum on the other side – and did being a midwife make it easier or harder?

After being a midwife for thirteen years, Devon felt like she knew a lot about women, pregnancy, labour, birthing and babies. She'd assisted hundreds of women and thought she'd been asked every question imaginable. She also thought she had the answers – evidence-based answers – and had supported women through a vast spectrum of birthing experiences.

'It wasn't until recently, when I became a mother for the first time, that I finally did my "practical" part of learning to be a midwife. I could previously only imagine what birthing, breastfeeding and mothering was actually like, though given my work and all that I'd witnessed, I didn't expect to find many surprises. I was, however, surprised by what surprised me!'

The first surprise came when Devon experienced morning sickness. Sickness that came all day, every day for four and a half months. Sickness that affected her ability to work, shop, cook, brush her teeth, lie down, sit up and eat. She knew morning sickness could be debilitating, but she suspects she hadn't truly appreciated the degree of its impact on women's lives before. No matter how much she tried her own advice – ginger tea, dry crackers, small meals – nothing worked like taking an antiemetic tablet. Medication is not usually the suggestion most promptly offered by a midwife, but Devon says, 'I wish I'd filled the script for Maxolon earlier!'

The second surprise came at her first ultrasound. She was 12 weeks and 4 days pregnant. She'd peed on a stick that showed two lines, had sore breasts and no period. She knew she was pregnant – she was a midwife – but without medical proof in the way of blood tests or an early ultrasound, there was always that shadow of doubt that maybe she was wrong. So when Devon saw her baby on the screen for the first time, she sobbed. It was just such a relief to see a baby in there. 'I don't know why my reaction surprised me, but I think having seen so many images of babies before, I thought this was just another ultrasound. As the saying goes, it's different when it's your own.'

The third surprise came when Devon arrived at 40 weeks and 12 days' gestation and still hadn't birthed. 'I never imagined that I would become impatient, but I discovered it really is challenging to not focus on the estimated due date. March 28 came and went. Suddenly I was 40+4, 40+8, 40+10, 40+12 . . .' All the times she'd sympathised with 'overdue' women, advising them to enjoy the quiet before the baby came; to rest, to see a movie, to have dinner out with their partner, to have a facial. Well, it turns out she'd already done all those things at 38 and 39 weeks, and so by the time D-day arrived, she really did feel well and truly cooked. Now she understands how exciting it is awaiting labour and the impatience you feel for the moment you finally meet your baby.

'I will still give the same advice to women in the future, but it'll be followed by, "I know how hard it is to be patient . . . I really do know."'

She also discovered she had to choose an induction of labour. Through her midwifery experience, she was well aware of the cascade of intervention, the concept that once medical intervention occurs, it is likely that further interventions will be required. If you interfere once, by breaking waters or putting in a drip, you have committed to having a baby. So, by hook or by crook, you have exponentially increased your chance of having to interfere again, with extra pain relief, the possibility of forceps or vacuum, or the increased risk of caesarean section. But as she approached the end date of 42 weeks, the pressure mounted and Devon was required to adjust her mindset to accept those risks. She had to frequently remind herself that many women who are induced do still enjoy a relatively natural and normal birth, despite that fact that the body wasn't the driving force to start the labour. She had to have faith that she too could keep things as normal as possible, but also be prepared for the unexpected.

Devon's fourth surprise came when out popped a boy after her twenty-hour induced labour, which she hadn't expected to take quite so long. Well, actually, the fourth surprise probably came a few hours earlier when he was declared a 'deflexed OP (occipito posterior)' baby; that is, facing the wrong way with his head back! This usually means a long labour and back pain for Mum. Devon had previously coached and supported many other women through 'back labour', often reported as incredibly difficult, excruciating and intolerable, and the intensity of her back pain lived up to other women's descriptions. So much so that after twelve hours of established labour, with a deflexed posterior baby and at 9 centimetres dilated, she asked for an epidural. This was also something that she never thought she would need or request.

'I was immensely grateful to my support team for supporting me in my choices.' With water immersion – one of Devon's passions, which she fought to offer birthing women at her hospital – no longer an option, gas no longer effective, and Devon losing the stamina and willpower to keep going, the epidural gave some relief for the final few hours of labour. This is when she remembered that especially in long labours, where exhaustion becomes a problem and the mum just needs to catch her breath, epidural anaesthetic comes into its own.

As long as it is an effective block, and numbness extends from your umbilicus to your feet, the contractions magically disappear from your radar and you can call time out. Thank goodness for that chance for a brief sleep, to rebuild your reserves and refocus on the end goal.

The respite did the trick and finally Felix was born. Devon hadn't found out what she was having, but after three vivid girl dreams, she was expecting a girl. Felix was a genuine, incredible surprise, and she was instantly smitten. She was also immensely thankful that her birth plan request to have immediate skin-to-skin with Felix was met, allowing those first precious moments of the hot, wet heaviness of her brand-new baby on her chest; and delayed cord clamping, so that the umbilical cord continued to supply Felix with oxygen and iron-rich blood for several minutes before it was clamped and cut.

As for parenting, Devon discovered this was a joy. Motherhood has exceeded all her expectations. Being a midwife had certainly prepared her for the day-to-day care of a baby, so she entered her new role confident in wrapping, swaddling, bathing, settling and breastfeeding. She felt confident in her ability to care for Felix and had been blessed with a charming and well-behaved baby. And, if you ask Devon, well, Felix is the best-looking, smartest, cutest, funniest and most loving of all the babies in the world. 'Yes, I have become one of those parents . . . Again, as I had been told, it's different when it's your own. It really is.' Babies rely on that natural adoration and guardianship to survive.

What has surprised Devon about parenting? Breastfeeding

really is fantastic. She has been lucky to have an easy breast-feeding experience that she attributes simply to her trust in the process, her big 4-kilogram baby with his big mouth, her 'designed for it' breasts and generous milk supply. She also allowed Felix to learn to self-attach from the very first feed – which meant just waiting for Felix to bounce around until he sniffed out the place he needed to be, and actually made his way there by himself.

Facilitating the opportunity for a baby to learn correct attachment at the first feed in that first hour of life, safe from interfering hands, just being observed, is one of the true joys of midwifery. Imagine unfocussd but wide eyes, that little pink tongue going in and out, those chubby fists opening and closing as he kneads his mother's breasts, the bobbing head swivelling as he blurrily scans the warm skin around him . . . suddenly spying that dark ring of areola skin around the nipple that Mother Nature has made incredibly enticing, a primitive urge has him wriggling and leaning until the breast and nipple is in exactly the right place. His mouth opens exactly as it should, because he's practised on his hands before this, and closes over his target. No damage for the mother, and bliss for baby.

The fact that we have finally stepped back from assuming babies need our help to learn one of the basic survival instincts in how to feed is one of the quiet advances spreading like sunlight through post-birth care. That, and ensuring a newborn baby doesn't go straight into bunny rugs but spends at the very least that first hour snug against the mother's skin between her breasts, as long as she and baby are well, or the dad's skin if the mum can't. Studies have proven that to warm a cold baby, skin-to-skin contact is faster and more precise than a humidic-rib or warm blanket, and that a mother's skin heats to the exact right temperature to warm her baby perfectly. And babies who have been acclimatised to the world in that first hour against their mother's skin adjust their breathing and heart rate faster and have the best chance of successful breastfeeding.

As Devon has found, it also means that even when she's half asleep at night, Felix can help himself to a snack in the dark.

With great relief, Devon has discovered that for her, inter-rupted sleep is not as difficult as she anticipated. She believes it helps if mothers can adjust their perception and expectations of sleep with a new baby. After years of watching mums on night duty, Devon didn't expect to sleep through the night, but instead takes into account all the snippets of sleep through-out the day. Being able to say to herself, 'I slept for eight hours today' sounds much better than 'I was awake every two or three hours last night to feed'.

So, would Devon change the way she cares for women dur-ing pregnancy, in labour and postnatally, now she's had Felix? Devon says no, because her philosophy of midwifery hasn't changed. That philosophy is providing women and their fam-ilies with evidence-based, holistic, women-centred maternity care. Devon has taken on board the research findings that women who are empowered and take control of their own care report feeling the most satisfaction with their birthing experi-ence. Whether women choose a drug-free birth or an epidural, whether they labour spontaneously or are induced, whether they birth vaginally or via caesarean section, and whether they choose to feed with breast milk or formula, she supports them in their choice.

The way women birth is not always entirely within their control. Many factors will influence the decisions made and the journey taken, but Devon believes every labour and birth can be an enriching experience for the mother. Education, support and remembering everyone's mutual goal enables a woman to achieve an amazing birth and nurtures her towards positive parenting.

Maternity education has always been Devon's particular area of interest within her midwifery career. Devon trained in Western Australia, like Mandy, and is currently employed as the midwifery educator at a hospital in northern NSW, a role that she relishes. She absolutely believes that doctors and midwives should participate in ongoing education together within the workplace, as they work as a team each day. Sharing their experiences and points of view enables better understanding of each other's roles and enhances mutual respect, which flows on to improvement in outcomes for women and babies. That is her passion and ultimate goal. 'I've been fortunate to be involved in a number of programs that foster the learning relationship between maternity care providers and can see just how beneficial it is for all involved.'

Before Felix was born Devon spent time managing the Northern Territory Simulation Lab on behalf of Flinders

Medical School, managing its day-to-day running, teaching, and creating educational programs. Devon found the most enjoyable sessions involved doctors, nurses and midwives from the anaesthetic, paediatric and obstetric departments, and the use of SimMom, a talking, breathing, birthing obstetric mannequin. SimMom can have a postpartum haemorrhage or an eclamptic fit, as well as giving learners the opportunity to deliver her baby, manage a shoulder dystocia (when the baby's shoulders have jammed against the mother's pubic bone; imagine broad shoulders fitting through a narrow doorway – some adjusting is required) or assist with a breech birth. A debrief takes place at the end of each obstetric scenario and is highly valuable in training staff in communication and teamwork, as well as clinical skills and management of obstetric emergencies.

Devon says it was always interesting to observe what others learnt from the simulations. Often it was the little things that had the biggest impact; for example, encountering an unfamiliar piece of equipment or protocol, or discovering how to escalate and call for assistance, or considering how a particular scenario might impact the woman and her family. There's no doubt that multidisciplinary simulation sessions are valuable for all involved, and Devon believes she's fortunate to share teaching opportunities as an instructor with ALSO, FONT and PROMPT (PRactical Obstetric Multi-Professional Training) courses around Australia.

Devon's most memorable training with SimMom took place in a dusty quarry outside of Darwin. The Sim Lab staff carted 70 kilograms' worth of SimMom, packed into two suit-cases, into a makeshift field hospital designed to train surgeons and nurses in first-line emergency response. The surgeons were very impressed with SimMom, as she enabled them to learn emergency vacuum extraction (where a flat plastic cup is placed on the baby's head and a vacuum suction holds it on so that when the mother has a contraction and pushes, the doctor can apply downward force on the handle of the cup to help the baby's head birth), perimortem caesarean section (delivery of a baby by a 'splash and slash' caesarean on the spot – usually not in an operating theatre) after a mother has been unable to be resuscitated and has no heartbeat after four minutes and shoulder dystocia and breech extraction. 'We are very lucky in Australia to be able to access such high-quality obstetric education where networking with colleagues is encouraged and embraced, and creativity and innovation within training is evident.'

Devon also has a passion for music. In 2003, while com-pleting her Postgraduate Diploma in Midwifery, she and her fellow grads were given their most challenging assessment task: to pick a topic in midwifery and to present it creatively as part of a university exhibition. Many in the class were terrified at the prospect of needing to be creative; they'd thought they were completing a science- and evidence-based degree, not a creative arts degree, and wondered at the rationale for such an assessment!

Devon, however, was excited. As a singer and pianist, this gave her the opportunity to join two areas of her life that she loved, and she planned to create a song about the beauty of birthing, about the bond between mother and child, and about the miracle of life. 'That was, until it was suggested that I instead choose a topic I was not comfortable with: grief and loss.'

As a student midwife, Devon was terrified at the prospect of caring for a bereaved family, but she took the advice and began her learning curve in the world of grief and loss. Coincidentally, it was at this time that someone close to her experienced a miscarriage at 11 weeks. Additionally, she reflected on her beloved grandmother, who had lost her firstborn son just twenty minutes after his birth. He had died of 'pure exhaustion', she was informed. This was sixty-five years ago. Not one photograph, handprint or footprint, or lock of hair exists of this little boy. Devon's grandfather was not present at the birth, and her grandmother did not get to see or hold her little baby. In the Catholic hospital where he was born, all babies who died were baptised either John or Mary, but he became known as Mark to Devon's grandparents. Devon remembers her family acknowledged Mark's birthday, and knew which star was his. Losing a child was clearly something one never forgot.

With these stories in mind, she wrote the song 'We Dreamed of You'. The lyrics and music just flowed, and before she knew it she was performing it at the end-of-semester exhibition. After the performance, a number of women came to share their stories with her. Multiple miscarriages, stillbirths, babies that died at birth or within their first few hours . . . Devon had no idea there were so many women who had experienced this loss. She was also asked if it was possible to purchase copies of her song . . . and this led to the song reaching an even wider audience after Devon had it professionally recorded, with her talented sister playing piano and singing backing vocals.

King Edward Memorial Hospital in Perth was the first hospital to provide a copy of 'We Dreamed of You' to women experiencing the loss of a baby. Other hospitals have followed suit. Over 2000 copies of 'We Dreamed of You' have now been given to families and Devon is grateful to know that, for many of them, the song has provided just a little comfort in their time of grief.

Naturally, then, perinatal loss is another area of midwifery for which Devon feels great empathy, and she believes she was incredibly fortunate to consolidate all she had learnt through her time working at King Edward Memorial Hospital. She's proud that Australian maternity services provide families with one-on-one midwifery care, and with mementoes that enable them to later reflect and pay tribute to their child.

So when Devon goes back to work after her maternity leave, what will her role be? As a midwifery educator, she has a varied work week. With her unit manager's support, each month she creates a schedule of education sessions to deliver and displays this in the midwives' station for all to see. This enables all staff, including doctors and students, to see what topics are coming up, and piques their interest to encourage attendance.

Session topics include vaginal examination, using a fantastic mannequin called 'Charlie and His Mum'; how to manage shoulder dystocia and vaginal breech using 'Sophie', another excellent birthing training model; waterbirth management, including how to remove a woman from the bath in an emergency. There are also perineal repair workshops using vaginas Devon made with foam from Bunnings, CTG reviews of real fetal heart patterns to discuss areas of potential confusion and subsequent management, and perinatal loss workshops, as well as sessions on an array of obstetric and neonatal emergencies. 'The midwives I work with are a dedicated and motivated bunch, who regularly attend education sessions and simulations, despite the busy work schedule.' Devon's plan is to deliver at least three sessions per week, though sometimes the workflow of the unit has other ideas.

As the clinical midwifery educator, Devon also attends real obstetric and neonatal emergencies. Her role is to support the staff in the birthing suite to take the lead in the emergency, but she is available to step in as required. She makes an excellent scribe, is an expert in weighing blood loss, and will support the support people until the crisis is over. Thankfully, most births are perfectly normal, but she admits she thrives on the adrenalin rush of obstetric emergencies and neonatal resuscitation.

Other duties include orientating new staff to the unit, attending staff development meetings, sitting in on interviews, working alongside staff who need extra support or who wish to begin working in a new area, and her favourite, working on the floor as a midwife when it is busy, which means at least once a fortnight she gets to help out in the birth suite. The beauty of busyness is that usually there are many labouring 'walk-ins', women who are labouring spontaneously and are ready for their one-to-one midwifery support. These are the labours and births Devon enjoys the most, as they usually involve the least intervention and are most likely to result in normal birth; the labours and births that she walks away from feeling inspired and in awe of the brilliance of women, their bodies, their families and their new babies. These are the days when Devon thanks her lucky stars that she was called to be a midwife.

Acknowledgements

So we come to the end of this book of midwifery stories and I hope you have enjoyed meeting the midwives, the mothers, and their families. For me it has increased my love of what I do and my admiration for midwives everywhere.

I had an inkling, but not full comprehension, of the scope that is covered by midwives in Australia. I can see now I have only scratched the surface of the wonderful stories that are touched on in this book. That fact only makes me more excited to search for more stories of midwives meeting mothers needs and perhaps stretch myself in new experiences in new places meeting new families as they birth.

I have to thank Andrea McNamara, who had the idea for this book several years ago and my apologies that it took so long for me to reach this point. You knew how much I would love and feel privileged to do this and you were right. Thank you, Andrea.

To dear Sarah Fairhall, my lovely editor and publisher at Penguin Random House, who has been so patient and supportive, thank you again. Thanks also to Jo Rosenberg for early input, Hilary Reynolds for the fabulous edits and copyedits, and Michelle Hamze photographer from Kempsey, (Broni was her midwife for her last baby and she took Broni's photo for the cover of the book which I thought was a lovely circle) and the fabulous art department at Penguin Random House for the cover.

To Clare Forster, my agent, from Curtis Brown, who has so much faith in me, loved the concept of this book from the beginning, and offers sage advice when I'm in need. You are just so savvy!

As always, my husband Ian, who offered to pay back the advance when it seemed I would never be able to do justice to this concept, though he may have offered because I was making his life hell. Thank you, my love, for helping me see instantly how much I wanted to meet this challenge.

To my writing family, all fabulous, but special mention to Trish Morey and Annie Seaton who put up their hands when I doubted I would get it done. To my midwifery and medical colleagues, in Kempsey and at ALSO, you are all champions, thank you.

But most of all I thank the midwives in this book, these busy, sleep-deprived, passionate midwives, for sharing intimate moments from their lives, and while maintaining privacy, sharing births with families who have touched them in so many ways. Theirs is a gift of caring for the women and families they serve and a gift in tenacity in striving to make it better.

From this journey I have discovered so much I was unaware of. I hope readers, young and older, are able to peer through the window into our world, and be amazed and touched, to appreciate a little of what midwives see, how much they care, and how important women and their families are to them.

And finally, I hope young women and men will read this book and consider taking on the gentle mantle of being a midwife to women. You could be a part of the new wave of caring and nurturing guardians of safety in birth and women's choice that is the way of the future and every woman's right.